April 27, 2006

Dr. Jeff —

May our good Lord shine on you for good health, happiness, & success forever.

Lynda Perugini

PHYSICAL & OCCUPATIONAL THERAPISTS' JOB SEARCH HANDBOOK

PHYSICAL & OCCUPATIONAL THERAPISTS' JOB SEARCH HANDBOOK

Your Complete Job Search Strategy:
How to Hire; How to Be Hired

by
Lynda Peringian, M.S., CPC

Therapy Careers Press, Inc.
Southfield, Michigan

Published by
Therapy Careers Press, Inc.
29451 Greenfield, Suite 112
Southfield, Michigan 48076

ISBN: 0-9622773-0-4
Library of Congress Catalog Card No.: 89-50592

Printed in the United States of America

Library of Congress Cataloging in Publication Data

Peringian, Lynda
    Physical & Occupational Therapists'
        Job Search Handbook

    Bibliography.
    Includes index.
    1. Physical Therapy-Job Search-United States.
    2. Occupational Therapy-Job Search-United States.

Dedication

To all the individuals who have been inspirational, and taught me about work: family, teachers, colleagues, students, clients, and other friends.

Table of Contents

Introduction 13

1. Taking Stock of Yourself 19
   Goals: Long and Short-Term; Before the Job Search;
   Self Evaluation; Risks and Gains; Geographical Con-
   siderations; Why Therapists Change Jobs; Therapist's
   Career Quiz

2. Developing a Plan of Action 35
   Preparation; The Unpublished Market; Networking;
   Professional Contacts; Friends; Conventions and
   Associations; Professional Publications; Answering
   Advertising; Employment Agencies

3. Creating Effective Tools 51
   Pointers for Cover Letters; Sample Cover Letters; How
   to Write a Resume That Sells Yourself; Sample
   Resumes—New Graduate and Experienced Therapists

4. The Interview 75
   Do Your Homework; Dressing to Get the Job; Travel-
   ing; Arriving on Time; The Waiting Room; the First In-
   terview Contact; Filling Out Application Forms; The
   Interview Conversation; Meals During Interviews;
   Positives and Negatives of Job Interviews; Interview
   Questions; Tricky Questions You Should Be Able to
   Answer; Telephone Manners and Test; Post-Interview
   Etiquette-Thank-You Letters

5. Through the Employer's Eyes 97
   Strategies of Staffing: Retention and Recruitment;
   Outline of Employee Concerns; Contracting Com-
   panies; Employing Physical and Occupational Therapy
   Assistants

6. The Employer's Administrative Functions 119
   The Selection Process—Six Stages: Screening, Rank-
   ing, Interviewing, Checking References, Making the
   Final Hiring Decision and Job Offer; Employer's Legal
   Requirements; Employee Orientation; Performance
   Reviews; Termination of Employment

7. Conclusion 143
   Post Search Networking and Self-Evaluation; Tips on
   Succeeding in Your New Job or Assignment; How to
   Get the Salary You Deserve; What to Do if Your New
   Job Isn't Working Out

   Appendix 155

              Job Search Checklist
              Salary Surveys
              Network Logs: Personal Contact, Phone,
                            Mail, Interview, Follow-
                            Up, Responses-Offers/
                            Acceptances/Rejections
              Resources/References
              Bibliography

   Index 175

Figures

Figure 1: Self Evaluation . . . . Chapter 1-27

Figure 2: Geographical Consideration . . . . . Chapter 1-30

Figure 3: Reasons Managers Change Jobs . . Chapter 1-32

Figure 4: Job Change Attractions . . . . Chapter 1-32

Figure 5: Therapist's Career Quiz . . . . Chapter 1-34

Figure 6: Resume Critique . . . . Chapter 3-65

Figure 7: Physical Therapy Practice
Settings . . . . Chapter 4-80

Figure 8: Types of Patients Occupational
Therapists Service . . . . Chapter 4-80

Figure 9: Application Form . . . . Chapter 4-85

Figure 10: Positives and Negatives of Job
Interviews . . . . Chapter 4-87

Figure 11: Traditional Organization Layout—
Rehabilitation Department . . . . . . Chapter 5-102

Figure 12: Modern Rehabilitation Department: Patient
and Family Centered Model . . . . . Chapter 5-103

Figure 13: Outline of Employee Concerns . . Chapter 5-114

Figure 14: Hospital Contract Management
Services . . . . Chapter 5-116

Figure 15: Characteristics of a Good
Interviewer . . . . Chapter 6-124

Figure 16: Pre-Employment Inquiry
Guide . . . . Chapter 6-134-137

Figure 17: Do's and Don'ts for Salary
Review . . . . Chapter 7-150

Figure 18: Job Change Timetable . . . . Chapter 7-154

Acknowledgments

This book would not have been possible without the help from others. I would like to thank the reviewers who assisted me with suggestions, accuracy, and encouragement:

Physical Therapists: George Andrews, PT; Roberta
                Cottman, PT; Raymond Lynch, PT;
                and Robert Mele, PT.
Occupational Therapists: Katie Goodwin, OTR;
                and Linda K. Katt; OTR.
Attorneys: Patrick J. Clarke, JD; Donald S. Skup-
                sky, JD; and Jerry J. Kaufman, JD.
Editors: Cely DeGracia, Dewey Little, and
                Kathleen McBroom.

Special thanks to my parents, Mike and Clara Peringian for their years of encouragement; my brother Charles Peringian for his interest; and Rev. V. Tootikian for initially suggesting me to write this book. My deepest appreciation goes to my sincere, long-term friend, Dewey Little, who has made many suggestions, been very supportive from the initial stages of the manuscript, and has helped keep it alive.

11

Introduction

A major issue in physical and occupational therapy today is the shortage of qualified therapists to meet an ever-increasing market demand. Present shortages of therapists have been fueled by a number of factors, such as legislation concerning the elderly—Medicare, Medicaid, and the Older American Act. Another factor is changes in today's health care delivery system: shorter hospital stays, a transition from institutional settings, and a growing complexity of health care options. Business and industry have realized that injury prevention programs can save money, and are turning to therapists to develop fitness, wellness and anti-injury programs. School systems have increased their need for therapists because of advanced screening evaluations and increases in treatment of handicapped children.

All these indicators point to a soaring need for therapy services as well as an increase in higher educational standards to train these professionals. According to a July 1988 study by the Institute of Medicine in Washington, D.C., the national population growth average is expected to be about 20 percent by the year 2000. Increased pediatric and maternal health programs will further strain the currently understaffed rehabilitation and health promotion services. Another consideration is that the number of severely disabled people, ages 17 to 44, has grown 400 percent in the past 25 years, according to the National Center of Health Statistics.

Occupational and physical therapists are two of the nation's fastest growing health care professions, according to the U.S. Department of Labor. Therapists can be employed in health clinics, fitness centers, day-care programs, holistic

13

health centers, hospitals, rehabilitation centers, schools, home care agencies, universities and colleges, and nursing homes. All of these facilities serve more than 32 million Americans, who suffer from all kinds of physical disabilities. Primary causes such as stroke, arthritis, back pain, birth defects, and catastrophic trauma involving brain and spinal cord damage further increases the demand. For example, the value of a therapist in promoting independence to the disabled by restoring a paralyzed limb to work again is a precious gift. The many valuable services therapists provide to our society make the physical and occupational therapists highly respected.

The *Occupational Outlook Handbook* reports employment opportunities for physical and occupational therapists will steadily increase through the mid-1900s due to the anticipated rapid acceleration of rehabilitation services. More lives are being saved as medical technology improves and as consumer awareness of medical services increases. At the same time, the increase of the elderly population stretches the already limited supply of qualified therapists.

Along with the obvious need for therapists comes the equally apparent question of how to recruit qualified personnel. The therapist grapples with the decision of choosing the "right position," while the employer confronts the problem of recruiting from a limited supply of qualified candidates. Both the employee and the employer want to be successful; this success can be achieved by knowing the ins and outs of simple good manners. Knowing the basic rules of etiquette enhances your ability to handle colleagues, clients, and superiors with tact and style. You create your image for better or for worse by the way you handle yourself.

Obviously, therapists change jobs for an endless variety of reasons. Some seek advancement opportunities, or increases in salary and bonuses, or new challenges and responsibilities or better working conditions. Many wish to relocate or are transferred, and others need to find a new position after losing a present one. Meanwhile, new graduates explore the job market enthusiastically, anxious to begin their careers.

For the newcomer and seasoned professional alike, one of the most difficult decisions is whether or not to accept a new position. It is human nature to prolong, procrastinate and simply avoid making a major decision. Taking steps to actually change jobs can be confusing and frightening. To ease that difficulty, this handbook presents guidelines for both the employee and the employer. No books that I have been able to discover have been written on the subject of the job search process for occupational and physical therapists. The information contained in this book, therefore, will give you a prospective in techniques to provide a successful search, whether you are an employee or employer. It is a "self-help" book and is designed as a textbook of reference to assist you now and in the future.

In the first four chapters we will concentrate on the employee, by examining goals, self evaluation, and developing a plan of action. We then will address creating effective cover letters and resumes and discuss the interview process. Questions the employee should be familiar with for the interview are covered, along with answers to tricky interview questions. The art of telephone manners, post-interview follow-up, how to get the salary you deserve, and suggestions to follow even if your new job is not working out are covered in Chapter 7. Meaningful guidelines concerning standards of behavior for both new graduates and experienced therapists, regardless of age, gender, or current employment status are presented.

The employer's side of the job search process is reviewed in Chapters 5 and 6. With the diminishing pool of physical and occupational therapists in the nineties and beyond, we will review twenty strategies for recruitment and retaining staff. Possible courses of action on staying on the competitive edge will provide insight and awareness to the employer. Other alternatives to staffing—contract companies and employing physical and occupational therapy assistants—are also suggested. The six stages of the selection process are presented so that the employer has an organized model to follow. The employer's legal requirements, employee orientation, performance reviews, and termination are discussed in order to effectively aid the employer in the administrative functions.

In this book both the employee and the employer can examine the job search process and become familiar with each other's point of view, which will lead to mutually beneficial relationships. This handbook will show the employee that it is possible to make the right career choices by employing the art of good manners, without burning your bridges, and even making friends along the way. Employers will improve their odds for success by reviewing the suggestions provided and broadening their knowledge. By studying and practicing the contents in this handbook, you can improve your situation, success, and happiness.

BON VOYAGE:
Physical and Occupational Therapists

I wish you the best of luck whether you are an employer seeking to hire therapists or you are a therapist looking for employment.

The aim of this book is to help you now and in the future and to give you guidelines and suggestions for a successful career.

Best wishes.

Taking Stock of Yourself

- Goals: Long-Term and Short-Term
- Before the Job Search
- Self-Evaluation
- Risks and Gains
- Geographical Considerations
- Why Therapists Change Jobs
- Therapists' Career Quiz

CHAPTER 1
Taking Stock of Yourself

In space travel, astronauts must hit a relatively small "launch window" through which light, heat and radio waves can penetrate. Likewise, in advancing your professional therapy career, you must access your own personal "launch window" with a precisely calculated plan.

From experience you know you can not always be in charge of everything, but on this mission your own importance ranks supreme. You are the only one who can take stock of yourself . . . and that is your initial task. It sounds simple, but it is not. Many factors can throw you off your course.

For example, imagine yourself right now in each one of the following scenarios:

• You are unemployed—fired, laid off, terminated, resigned, or a recent graduate.
• You have been offered a different position in the same company—a promotion, demotion or lateral move.
• You are happily employed, and you are offered another interesting position elsewhere.

Whatever your situation, the time will come when you must reset your goals and do a little soul searching . . . my imperative is Study Yourself! Determine what you want for tomorrow. For instance, your goals as a student in physical or occupational therapy are no more likely to remain constant over a five or ten year span than is the weather. Both goals and the weather are based on constantly changing data and both possess what Samuel Clemens called "dazzling uncertainty." Some of that uncertainty can be removed by planning, but some students tend to be shortsighted when it comes to career planning. They typically dream only of graduation and the end of a rigorous training program.

21

On the other side of the career pendulum, the experienced therapist often gets caught in the web of daily tasks and does not take time to contemplate their five or ten year goals. All things change—especially your situation. Many staff therapists find the job that once satisfied their financial needs, but it no longer matches their needs or desires because their career goals have shifted. Someone once said:

"If needs matched desires,
We'd all ride wooden tires
And forego the wheels
Of modern automobiles. "

Goals: Long-Term and Short-Term

When you plan your goals, you must identify the skills required for the job. Along with the necessary skills, do you also have the desire to do the work? It is also important to consider desire-type factors such as: personal fulfillment, family, intellectual challenge, physical needs and financial security.

The opportunities and roles of a therapist can be many and varied, so whatever you elect to do must match these goals.

Make a list of immediate goals. Write them down just as you would for a college assignment. It will be a written itinerary for a trip that most people plan but few people follow.

Perhaps your family or personal goal now is to move to a larger home. This is an important goal; do not discount it. Include it with your other short-term goals, and give each one a rating of one to ten.

On the short-term side, a career goal may be to gain management experience in a hospital. Then combine your short and long-term goals as follows:

• On a personal level, perhaps you want to retire financially comfortable at age 62 and travel with your spouse. Or perhaps your children will need college tuition.

• With regards to a career, you may want to own your own private practice to carry on your work and your name.

The important thing is to identify what you want to do as a therapist as early as possible. The next decision involves making the right choice in employment.

Before the Job Search

It is easy to grumble, feel dissatisfied, and think that you are in a rut. Most therapists have such feelings, even experienced department heads. However, a job change is not always the best answer.

Take a long look at the specific reasons you are dissatisfied, and evaluate those reasons along with an honest appraisal of what is satisfying about your present position. Remember, something attracted you to your current job in the first place.

Many people change positions only to discover they have not changed the basic unhappiness they feel about their work. So they decide to change again. This can lead to a reputation as a job-hopper, and raise employer questions about loyalty which can lower your opportunities for employment.

Therefore, before you search for a new position, consult with selected confidents and others who might shed light on your concerns. These people can come from both within and outside of your workplace. For example, you might want to try the following plan of action:

- Discuss your problems, interests, and concerns with your spouse, trusted relatives—away from the job.
- Talk with your superior, if possible. Ask, "What can we do to solve the problem and make the department run more smoothly?"
- Ask your co-workers about their problems and see if they match yours. You could find out that the problem is not yours alone, or that you, perhaps, are part of the problem.
- Check with other therapists in similar facilities to determine if the problem or concerns are widespread, and if similar problems do exist, what positive actions are being taken?
- Arrange a confidential meeting with your superior and

his or her boss to explain your concerns, if you believe this might be an acceptable move. If politically unwise, completely avoid it.

Now, evaluate your relationship with your employer by asking yourself questions such as:

• If you have been told to be patient and wait for changes, and you have waited for months or years, is it possible that these changes will ever come?

• Are you prepared to lose your job, if your employer finds out that you are looking for another opportunity?

• Is there a possibility for a promotion or can you transfer to another area and will this solve your problems?

• Have you been receptive to suggestions on ways to improve these problems? What actions have been taken to make your job better?

• If you decide to stay, can you let go of your feelings of dissatisfaction? Can you and are you perceived as a positive worker rather than a complainer?

After you consider these factors, you still may decide that you want a job change. Nobody wants to deal with an unhappy worker, and you certainly do not want to join the ranks of the disenchanted—especially since therapists have so much to offer!

Self-Evaluation

Evaluate your job goals and objectives by taking a few minutes and take stock of your strengths and weaknesses. See Figure 1: Self-Evaluation. This may not be the easiest task you have ever done, but it is not the toughest either. Just ask yourself, "What are my therapy skills and strengths?" and "What do I enjoy most in therapy?" Areas of excellence and enjoyment often coincide.

Rate yourself on the following traits. These traits are seen as strengths and are highly valued by employers in physical and occupational therapy:

24

Strengths

• Leadership—a professional therapist needs to be a path-finder, not simply a path-follower.

• Receptive Learner—the ability to quickly absorb new knowledge and techniques is essential.

• People Skills—patients require a great deal of understanding and support; so do colleagues.

• Quality Oriented—when it comes to health care, nothing can replace a concern for the highest quality.

• Risk Taker—no one ever solved a problem without taking some risk, and therapists are problem solvers.

• Economical and Practical—keeping an employer economically solvent is not just the employer's problem, but the staff's problem, too.

• Negotiator—a calm, reasonable approach settles most differences.

• Personal Appearance—cleanliness and neatness ranks high on the want list of most employers.

Now let us see if you recognize any weaknesses that might "turn-off" potential employers. Some of the most dismaying shortcomings found in therapists, according to their employers, include the following:

Weaknesses

• Impulsive—not using your head to solve problems is contraindicated, because that shows immaturity.

• Late or Never on Time—this cardinal sin indicates decreased interest and motivation.

• Overbearing—knowledge comes in through the senses and by being receptive to your surroundings. Therefore, listening to others pays off more than talking.

• Messiness and Untidiness—this is not a virtue, but a cross that parents bear; employers usually are not that tolerant.

• Following and Never Leading—reach out for the best you can be. Life is like being on a dog sled team, where the scenery only changes for the lead dogs.

• Exceeding Your Budget—often the worst thing anyone

can try to do to solve a problem by overspending unnecessarily.

- Too Bossy—to over-dictate and over-control people causes discontent and rapport.

- Compromiser—settling for differences that are against your values shows weakness. Your ideas and points of views need attention and work.

Coming to grips with yourself as a person does not mean that you are God's gift to therapy because you have certain strengths, or that you are hopeless because you have weaknesses. Obviously, everyone has both. But you have an advantage in the job market if you can identify your character and make use of that knowledge. Perhaps you are failing to maximize your strengths by settling for less than you deserve. Perhaps your weaknesses are causing you problems. For example, you may need more management training to attain your goals. Identify your weak areas, and then take steps to strengthen them.

Now comes the time for soul-searching. "What do I want to be when I grow up?" Most people ask that question more than once during a lifetime. It is best to ask early on . . . and then keep on asking from time to time, because we all appear to have considerable amounts of Peter Pan in us.

Some of the questions that a soul-searching therapist might ask are:

- What do I want to accomplish in my business and personal life?
- Do I want to be a manager or a staff therapist?
- Do I enjoy working in small or large facilities?
- Do I like being a specialist or having broad responsibilities?
- Do I like to travel, spend overtime, or work long hours on the job?
- Do I want to live in a major city, a suburban area, or in the country?
- In what region of the United States would I like to live?
- Am I willing to relocate or do I want to stay put?

Figure 1: **Self Evaluation**

RATE YOURSELF

Strengths

- Leadership
- Fast learner
- Rapport with people
- High-quality oriented
- Risk taker
- Economical and practical
- Negotiator
- Clean and neat

Weaknesses

- Impulsive
- Late or never on time
- Overbearing
- Messy and untidy
- Follower, not a leader
- Gambler, spender
- Too bossy
- Compromiser

STRENGTHS:

1. _____
2. _____
3. _____
4. _____
5. _____
6. _____
7. _____
8. _____
9. _____
10. _____

WEAKNESSES:

1. _____
2. _____
3. _____
4. _____
5. _____
6. _____
7. _____
8. _____
9. _____
10. _____

Risks and Gains

Write down the advantages and disadvantages of both your present job and the new jobs you are considering. This will help you evaluate if you are gaining enough or risking too much.

Advantages might include such factors as:

- Convenient geographical location
- Competitive salary
- Well-known rehabilitation facility
- Good physical working conditions, including modern, state of the art equipment.

Disadvantages, for example, could be:

- Inadequate salary
- Non-progressive rehabilitation department
- Caseload of patients comprised of one type, with little or no variety.

Personalize the advantages and disadvantages. Your career choice does not have to be a gamble if you weigh the odds for success. If your advantages outweigh your disadvantages, then consider a change. Otherwise, why bother?

Let's look at a specific situation. You are a 33 year old physical therapist with a Masters in Public Health. You have been with a large hospital for seven years and have held three different positions.

Your potential growth in your current position is limited, and you have been offered a position with a smaller rehabilitation facility. This position will involve a lot of pressure and you are uncertain about how it will work out—however, it could advance your career.

If you take the job and it does not work out after a year or two, you still have the seven years of experience you had at the prior position in the large hospital. You now have experience in both large and small departments and you can go either way in your next position.

You will maintain a record of success without the reputation of excessive job-hopping, and the advantage of taking the job in the small rehabilitation facility may be a positive gain for your future career objectives.

Geographical Considerations

You may have restrictions on your ability to move. For example, if your spouse is happy and doing well, or your children are in school, you may not want to relocate.

Let us look at another situation. You have been offered a job that involves a big salary gain, but it is at a hospital on the other side of the country. The negative side is that if it does not work out, you have already moved your family. However, if you are 55 years old and statistics are working against you, it may be a good opportunity. The risks may be well worthwhile in this case. It is important to weigh positive gains against negative risks.

Some therapists have been driven to go wherever the best job seems to be. Before you sally forth, determine if the job's geographical location is compatible with your lifestyle today, and in five or ten years from now.

Moving to a job in another location is always expensive. To keep costs down make use of your home-town advantage. Begin your job search within your home area—where you know more people and they know you. Progressively, you might need to widen your search, to your home state, then to a group of surrounding states, and finally to the entire country. (See Figure 2: Geographical Considerations.)

Besides the immediate cost of moving, you must evaluate the new locale in terms of cost-of-living, schools, housing, mass transit, taxes and purchasing power. Also consider the effect the move will have on your family.

Another consideration for you as a therapist is whether the new area has an excellent reputation as a health center. Working at the only therapy facility in town may be rewarding in terms of breadth of service, but it can be limiting to your long-range career plans.

Not to be overlooked is any assistance your prospective employer will provide you with a complete relocation package.

Figure 2: **Geographical Considerations**

1. Search within your home area
2. Search within your home state
3. Search within a group of states
4. Search within the United States
5. Search in other countries

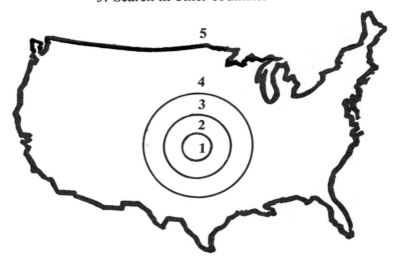

Why Therapists Change Jobs

It could be helpful to look at the reasons therapists leave their positions. The most common reasons reported by the Professional Advisory Council of the National Easter Seal Society, in their 1988 publication, *Crisis Ahead* were:

- Higher salary and benefits offered elsewhere
- Desire to continue on an advanced degree
- Desire by women to marry or have children
- Pursuit of administrative career or other career entirely

Respondents in one survey (see Figures 3 and 4: *Michigan Health Educator, 1980*), were asked to review a list of job-related factors and identify those most important to them. Over a thousand managers in thirty major cities across the country were polled. The three factors which emerged as most important were:

1. Possibility of advancement (96%)
2. Salary (83%)
3. Facility reputation among peers (80%)

Respondents were then asked to list the most compelling reasons for leaving a position. The five reasons most often given were:

1. No advancement opportunity (57%)
2. Poor management (39%)
3. Salary/bonus problems (38%)
4. Lack of challenge (24%)
5. Undesirable relocation (19%)

They were also asked to name the elements most important to them when considering relocation sites. The four factors most often cited were:

1. Recreational and cultural facilities (55%)
2. Lifestyle/environment (47%)
3. Climate (37%)
4. Job related factors (30%)

Interestingly, both the cost of living and the size of city ranked low on the list of importance.

Expectations about the new jobs were consistent with the reasons cited for leaving jobs. In order of frequency, they were:

1. Advancement opportunities
2. Salary and bonuses
3. Challenges and responsibilities
4. Working conditions (people, job, and environment)

This gives you some insight into what others consider when they make a job change decision.

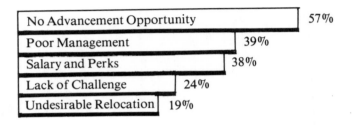

Figure 3: **Reasons Managers Change Jobs**

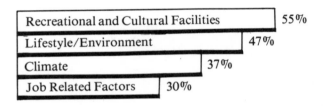

Figure 4: **Job Change Attractions**

Source: *Michigan Health Educator*
        Peringian, L., and Skeegan, S., June '80,
        Vol. 6, No. 3, 11-12

By taking stock of your present situation, you may find the person that you want to be. Following your self-evaluation, study and develop new goals and objectives. See Figure 5: Therapist's Career Quiz. Take a few minutes to quiz yourself and then score yourself. Which of these questions do you follow?

1. Do I need to develop new goals and objectives?
2. Do I consider myself happy at my present job?

This introspection and research may be frustrating for you at times, but it will be a rewarding experience.

Set a date for making a decision about whether or not to change jobs. Try to work through the tough times and resolve your present problems. However, if you decide to seek another position, do it while you are still employed.

Deciding whether to accept a new job offer is one of the most difficult decisions people face today in their careers. Making the decision may be frightening and difficult, but it should not be decided by a toss of a coin. Following the suggestions and guidelines in this handbook should guide you towards the right decision.

	Almost never	Rarely	Sometimes	Often	Almost always
Figure 5: Therapist's Career Quiz Peringian, L.					
1. I like to discuss my job as a therapist with my family and friends					
2. My job seems boring to me					
3. Co-workers seem encouraged by my positive attitude					
4. I know my strengths and weaknesses at work					
5. I do not like my co-workers, patients and superiors					
6. My work is exciting					
7. I read about therapy job opportunities and careers					
8. I receive compliments on my work					
9. I work overtime or volunteer because I enjoy doing it					
10. I do not like going in to work					
11. I get ideas about other careers by my hobbies and interests					
12. My work is suitable for me					

SCORING	INTERPRETATIONS

SCORING

Mark points in the spaces below and then add to totals in the column. Use the following point scale:

Almost never 1
Rarely 2
Sometimes 3
Often 4
Almost always 5

D scale	**R scale**
Question	Question
#2	#1
#5	#7
#10	#11

M scale	**C scale**
Question	Question
#3	#4
#6	#8
#9	#12

INTERPRETATIONS

Feelings

D scale = displeased   M scale = modernize
R scale = research   C scale = condense

1. If your D scale is higher than your R scale you may need to develop new goals and objectives.
2. If your D and C scales both are higher than your R and M scales you may need to develop new goals and objectives.
3. If your R scale is the highest you may need to develop new goals and objectives.
4. If your M and C scales are the highest you should consider yourself happy.

CHAPTER 2
Developing a Plan of Action

- Preparation
- The Unpublished Market
- Networking
- Professional Contacts
- Friends
- Conventions and Associations
- Professional Publications
- Answering Advertisements
- Using Employment Agencies

CHAPTER 2
Developing a Plan of Action

To plan but not to act is a shame; to act without a plan can result in disaster. When General George Custer fought the Sioux Indians at the Little Big Horn, he told his men, "We've got them." Apparently, much to his dismay, he was wrong.

In order not to meet a similar fate, you must plan your career in physical or occupational therapy, and then you can prepare to take action.

Preparation

You should develop a plan of action for your job search before any need or emergency exists. Remember that many therapy departments tend to be a little slower in late November and during the winter months. Remember too, that some facilities begin their search during January for additional positions that have been authorized by their new annual budgets. However, if you are serious, you should plan to start hunting immediately, without any special concern about the season, the state of the economy, or other extenuating factors.

Before you start your personal marketing plan, you must place your job campaign at the top of your personal priorities and develop a positive mental framework. A basic rule for job seekers is to remember the lyrics written by Harold Arlen and Johnny Mercer in 1945, which were made popular by Bing Crosby:

> *"You've got to ac-cent-u-ate the positive,*
> *e-lim-i-nate the negative,*
> *and don't mess with the mister in between."*

This kind of enthusiasm and energy . . . the big "E Factor" . . . must be an important element of your job search. Demonstrate that you are a winner, and that you have the energy to tackle anything. Show some passion for your profession. Many times qualified therapists do not get an offer because they convey negative feelings to the employer. This can be true of a new graduate or an experienced therapist.

Before you start your campaign, devise your action plan to include specific steps. The job market for therapists is constantly changing, just like Heraclitus' stream. Do not dangle your toes in the stream until you look inward and make the following assessments:

1. Review your strengths and weaknesses, your likes and dislikes, and your specific feeling towards job satisfaction requirements and goals. Include salary and benefit objectives. Identify your accomplishments and achievements as a therapist.

2. Identify the positions that are of interest to you, and the reasons why.

3. Establish a time schedule for your search, and then allocate sufficient time to accomplish it. Set a realistic completion date and revise as needed.

4. Organize your resume and review it. Have it neatly typed by a professional and keep it current, even if you have not changed jobs or are not actively looking for a job.

5. Prepare your cover letter; but no "cutesy" stuff. Keep it straightforward and businesslike, and keep the length to one page. Why shoot yourself in the foot before you get your foot in the door?

6. Develop a list of telephone numbers and addresses of individuals for future contacts.

7. Cultivate new business contacts and renew previous business and personal contacts.

8. Check your references; employers will. Make sure your personal and professional references are up to date, and remind these people that they are on your list of references and may be called upon.

9. Review geographical areas you would consider. Talk to your spouse, family and close friends. Consider the impact of relocation.

10. Consult all media for job openings advertising:

A. Physical Therapy:

> *Journal of the American Physical Therapy Association*
> *Today's Student Physical Therapist*
> *Physical Therapy Bulletin*
> *Physical Therapy Forum*

B. Occupational Therapy:

> *Occupational Therapy Week*
> *Occupational Therapy Forum*

C. Both Physical and Occupational Therapy:

> *Hospitals*
> *Physical Therapy/Occupational Therapy Job News*
> Association newsletters—national, state, district and section

Your local public library has a wealth of information, and provides newspapers and journals for out-of-town areas. (See Appendix for References and Resources.)

In order to be successful, getting your job action plan ready must command first attention. Be careful not to create any negative factors that employers would not want to hear. For example, you should do everything possible to assure that you are never without a current position. Those who hire do not add new employees to the workforce as an act of mercy. You are more desirable to them if you are presently employed.

This means that you should maintain good relations with your current and any past employers, if possible. Do not burn your bridges; always leave on the best of terms. Prospective employers will often look at your last employment as a critical reference.

A major mistake is to make job changes too often. Jumps from eight months at one facility to seven months at another can hinder you in your job search.

To keep your progress moving smoothly, remember not to promise more than you can deliver.

The Unpublished Market

The job market for the physical and occupational therapist is often hidden in an unpublished market . . . an invisible market. This hidden market includes jobs which will soon be available due to increases in staff, relocations, retirements, or other reasons.

The general public never hears about these openings because they are often filled from within the facility or through personal contacts. Many times the employers only post the vacancies on their bulletin boards so the employees have the first opportunity to apply. This way the employer saves time and money by not advertising and can hire and promote from within the facility.

Jobs that can not be filled from within may be advertised, but many are not. Never assume that all jobs are advertised. Even if no opening has been posted or advertised, it makes sense to apply for a job at a place where you believe you would like to work. Address your application directly to the Director of Occupational or Physical Therapy Department. Personnel directors are nice enough people, but therapy directors are the ones who hire the therapists.

Here is an example of how this "Invisible Market" works: John Smith, Director of Rehabilitation for XYZ Hospital, meets Doreen Jones, Director of Rehabilitation for ABC Hospital, at a professional meeting. During the lunch break, Doreen mentions that one of her staff is relocating and she will need to look for a replacement. John tells Doreen that he has a friend who happens to be looking for a position in Doreen's location and they exchange business cards. A few days later, John's friend goes for an interview and is offered the position.

Examples of the "visible" job market can be found by looking at newspaper ads, or by going to employment agencies, professional associations, or college placement services. These job listings are important, but you should make sure that you are accessing both the visible and the invisible markets.

In order to uncover the hidden, or unpublished job market, you need to use all of your contacts—both business associates and acquaintances. They will help you uncover the hidden market. You also need to employ good marketing skills, such as an effective direct mail campaign that includes a good resume and a well written cover letter. The hidden job market can also be accessed by using effective follow-up techniques and networking.

Networking

Since the beginning of the 1981 recession, networking has been very popular. It is not a new concept, but rather a reaffirmation that people in business really do need each other.

Networking is the development and use of business contacts to create a valuable body of information; in this case, prospective employers or employees. This involves putting together a personal network of professional contacts and acquaintances. You may want to appear at professional clubs and associations to increase your visibility.

Stay in touch with people and let them know that you are preparing to make a career move, and do not forget to follow-up. Your professional contacts should include a wide variety of resource people.

Professional Contacts

Therapists should include the following types of resource people in their professional contacts:

- Accountants
- Bankers
- Colleagues
- Consultants
- Dentists
- Doctors
- Lawyers
- Librarians
- Past Employers
- Political Associates
- Professional Recruiters
- Public Relations Contacts
- Sales Professionals and Suppliers
- Support Staff (Secretaries, Receptionists, etc.)

41

Remember the people in housekeeping, maintenance and other departments within your facility, too. If they are part of the grapevine, they are probably aware of what is happening there and within other health care facilities in the area.

Friends

There are few times when you have greater need to gather up your friends than during a job search. The task is not easy, but like Sisyphus of Greek mythology, you will have to keep pushing that rock up the hill. However, unlike Sisyphus your task will end and you will find a job. It will be easier if you count on friends such as:

- Acquaintances
- Neighbors at home and at work
- Past co-workers
- Relatives and their friends
- School friends and alumni

(See Appendix for Personal Contacts Log.)

Conventions and Associations

An excellent way to develop job leads and interviews is to attend conventions, workshops, regional meetings, seminars, continuing education meetings and medical meetings. Employers find that often the brightest therapists with the greatest potential participate in such activities. You will meet new colleagues and be exposed to many professional situations . . . both of which are very valuable in helping you to reach your career goals.

Both the American Physical Therapy Association and the American Occupational Therapy Association hold national conventions each year. A private practice section or another special section group can provide good opportunities for networking. These groups also have state and local associations that can help you and these organizations provide excellent opportunities to meet colleagues who can and will help you.

Usually, when you join one of these organizations you will receive a membership list including names, addresses, phone numbers of the very people you might want to contact regarding employment. Beyond that, you should attend all conventions and always take your resume with you, as this can provide you with excellent interview opportunities.

Be an active participant in the groups. Most associations exist thanks only to the support of volunteers to provide administrative and service assistance for committees. By helping out, you contribute a valuable service to your profession, display leadership skills . . . and gain important job contacts! This demonstrates the big "E"—Energy and Enthusiasm—for your profession, and employers look favorably on this quality.

Some of the clubs and associations you should consider as contact-productive include the following:

- Alumni groups
- Community organizations
- Professional associations
  (national, state and local)
- Public service groups
- Religious groups
- Social clubs
- Sporting clubs

Networking involves meeting people both formally and informally. Hopefully, you will develop rapport with your contacts and learn of word-of-mouth job opportunities.

Start with your professional contacts and simply ask them (in confidence) if they know of any positions available that fit your career objectives. Each person that you contact has a circle of friends, relatives and contacts, which means that additional help can occur from the most unexpected sources.

As you gain more experience with your contacts, continue on your list of friends, clubs, and association members. With practice, you can become an expert networker.

Be prepared for some disappointments, but do not be dismayed by rejection from some of the people you contact. On the bright side, remember that there are people who will become your real friends and who will stay with you long after you complete your search and locate your new position.

Professional Publications

Physical and occupational therapy publications contain a lot of information regarding your career field. Do not read

43

only the classified ad section, but read the entire publication. Many times you will find announcements of appointments of key personnel and other member news. You will find listings of projects, meetings, and conventions as well as the names of persons conducting these meetings. This is valuable because it will provide you with specific names and other information that will better prepare you for interviews.

Questions concerning current issues in therapy are common in job interviews. In physical therapy, you can learn about current clinical and management issues by reading professional publications. For example, *Clinical Management,* published by the American Physical Therapy Association, has presented articles on the job market as well as tips to help the employer attract the best qualified people. Keep in mind the importance of technical articles, found in such publications as *Journal of the American Physical Therapy Association.* Similarly, occupational therapists can find valuable reference material in the *American Journal of Occupational Therapy.*

In addition to reading such publications, try writing an article directed towards your professional peers. If you can get an article published, it will help you to become more visible in your field. This will highlight your knowledge and skills in a way that most employers find impressive. Never become discouraged in the attempt to be published; keep trying and regard it as a positive step in your career progression. Attitude changes everything! For example, some people shudder at the wail of an ambulance siren; others are relieved that someone is getting help. It is all a matter of attitude.

The advertising found in these professional publications also keeps you abreast of new therapy products and services. Such awareness of these developments will make you more valuable to employers. Research projects are also announced in the publications, along with grant monies allocated for research. This knowledge may be pivotal for therapists seeking jobs in research or in faculty positions.

Answering Advertisements

Newspaper or magazine advertisings are not always valid leads for jobs. They may provide a kind of map as to what is going on in your field. However, the actual amount of assistance offered can be compared to a classic story of a tourist seeking directions in rural New England:

"Where does this road go?" he asked.

"Can't say I'd ever seen it go nowheres," says the taciturn Yankee.

"Well how far is it to the next town?"

"Can't say. Never measured it."

"You're not very smart, are you?"

"Maybe not . . . but I ain't lost."

The point is that while you are job seeking, you are the one who is "lost," and you should not expect to get all of your answers in one place. Some employers advertise because they are unhappy with someone and want to "shake the tree" to see what they can find. However, often the advertisements are for real jobs, and thousands of therapists have obtained their positions through this means.

The Classified Section in Sunday newspapers are most widely used by employers and read by job seekers. That comes as no surprise. But, while you are in the job market, do not ignore advertisements in the weekday papers. These can include those placed by employers (sometimes blind ads —ads which do not list the employer's name but use a box number) as well as listings with recruitment firms.

Advertisements come in a variety of forms, and you should deal with each type separately. Consider the following categories:

1) *Hard to understand advertisements.* After reading the advertisement, you still do not understand what they want. The best thing to do is to phone them and find out what they want, providing there is a name or phone number.

2) *Misleading advertising.* They seem glamourous but really involve more work than it appears. For example, an advertisement seeking a chief physical therapist may sound

like a management position, but in reality you may find that you would be the only therapist, and you would be treating all patients and running the department with no plans in place to hire additional staff. Make sure the position is as good as it sounds.

3) *Advertisements that say nothing.* For example: "Physical Therapy Opening" or "Occupational Therapy Opening." You have no idea what is involved. You have to find out more by calling or writing.

4) *One-Way Advertisements.* They tell the requirements for the job, but none of the benefits. If you fill the requirements, be sure to find out what the benefits are during the interview. Otherwise, you are negotiating for unknown quantities. Do not neglect or ignore your objectives and priorities.

5) *Advertisements that do not identify the employer.* That may seem unfair to you. For all you know, the employer who asks that you reply to a blind box address may be your present employer. He or she may even be trying to replace you! But why place an unfair advantage in the employer's court? Understand, we are not trying to play sides, because we are all in this job-search/job-hire situation together. One answer to the "blind ad" is to have a friend answer it. Your friend can omit your name and any contact information or place of employment. Here is an example letter:

Dear Box Number 10:

I have a friend who matches your description for a "Supervisor of Out-Patient Therapy." This person has:
  —5 years clinical experience in an out-patient clinic
  —interest in a supervisory position
  —excellent rapport with people
  —can meet your salary offer

I have been asked to reply to you in confidence and will keep all communications confidential. There are no fees for my help and I can be reached at (313) 555-0000.

Sincerely,
Janis Baker

When you do respond to an advertisement, include a cover letter and a resume. Take care with a one page, straight-forward cover letter.

Keep copies of all advertisements that you respond to and notes of when you sent a resume. If you do get a response, you will have the specific advertisement to refer to. This will enable you to reply appropriately. (Also see Chapter 5—pages 109-110: employer's advertising campaign.)

Employment Agencies

Professional recruiters are often used by institutions to help recruit therapists and other personnel. Employment agencies offer a wide assortment of employment services, and are available for entry-level positions through advanced management positions. These agencies are regulated by laws in most states, and collect their fees from the employer.

If you choose to work with an agency, make sure you are comfortable with them and that they are specialists in working with physical and occupational therapists. A good agency can save you time and expose you to openings they know about from the inside track. Because you pay no fees, the agency can be a good addition to your search. A qualified agent will do a lot of legwork and research in helping you find the right job.

At the same time, be aware that an experienced recruiter will not work with you under the following conditions:

1) You have unrealistic expectations about the salary or the job you are seeking
2) Your employment history is very unstable or you are a constant job-hopper
3) You are found to be dishonest
4) You are attempting to make a counter offer to your current employer

There are two types of professional recruiters—the contingency recruiter and the retained recruiter. Contingency recruiters work on recruitment assignments—usually lower to middle level management positions, and incur payment only if their candidate is selected. There are no fees for candidates.

The retained recruiter has an exclusive arrangement with their clients and are usually looking for candidates for positions in middle or senior management levels. The retained agent receives a fee from the employer. The recruiter helps create the job descriptions, reviews the salary package and makes notes of strengths and weaknesses of the candidates.

Some facts about employment agencies worth noting include the following:

• Many employers do use agencies to fill their openings, and these positions are not advertised by the employer. Often employers will contact agencies to screen out people as well.

• There are no fees to applicants, usually; employers pay the fees. The fees are usually tax deductible and may be considered as an allowable direct cost, subject to the institution's reimbursement schedule.

• The agency keeps all communication confidential. You are told the name of the employer before you are referred.

• The recruiter will work with you to improve your resume and interviewing skills.

• You can receive information helpful for interview situations and with regard to prospective employers.

• You can be exposed to many openings, not just one opportunity.

• An experienced recruiter will work only those candidates they feel they can place and not all applicants. They can generally determine which candidates will be the easiest to place.

• A recruiter who specializes in only physical and occupational therapists can serve you better by his or her expertise in the field, rather than a generalist who may not have as many openings available for you.

• Agencies can give you fast post-interview follow-up information.

• Agencies can assist you in relocation, and they have access to out-of-town openings that you may have a hard time locating by yourself.

• There are good and honest recruiters and there are dishonest recruiters, just as there are good people and there are dishonest people. You can say the same rule for employers—bad and good. It is your decision to decide if you are comfortable working with a recruiter, but remember the same is true for the recruiter, whom is working for you at no cost to you. If the recruiter does not like your attitude, he or she can decide not to help you, and you may not receive any phone calls.

Creating Effective Tools

- Pointers for Cover Letters

- Sample Cover Letters
  1) To a target facility without a resume
  2) To a friend—no resume
  3) Letter with reference and resume
  4) Network letter using a bridge with a resume
  5) With resume to former associate
  6) New graduate to target facility
  7) Experienced therapist to target facility
  8) For mailing a resume to a recruiter
  9) Student seeking summer job—no resume

- How to Write a Resume That Sells Yourself

- Sample Resumes
  1) New graduate—physical therapist
  2) Experienced physical therapist
  3) New graduate—occupational therapist
  4) Experienced occupational therapist

CHAPTER 3
Creating Effective Tools

Preparing the right application package to present yourself at your best requires that you are at the helm. Certainly you can get assistance to avoid pitfalls, but ultimately you are selling a product that no one knows as well as you do.

Back in the 1940s and 1950s a talented sales consultant, Elmer Wheller, stormed the country with some memorable advice . . . "Sell the sizzle, not the steak!" Obviously sizzle is what people buy; they buy the benefits of what the product or service can do for them.

As a therapist seeking a job, you are the product . . . and what you offer to the employer is of primary importance. To begin with, your basic tools are the cover letter and the resume. For an entry level therapist, the cover letter is more important than the resume.

Pointers for Cover Letters

Always include a cover letter with your resume, whether you are applying for a first job or a tenth job. It will introduce you and serve as a summary of what skills you have to offer to the employer. Be sure to state your qualifications from the employer's viewpoint.

Here are some tips on drafting your cover letters:

1) Send your cover letter and resume to the department you wish to work for, rather than to the personnel department unless you are answering an advertisement that specifies replies to personnel. If you are seeking a director's position, send your application package to the administrator of the facility, unless specified otherwise by the advertisement.

2) Address your letter to a specific person, not a title. Take the time to find out the person's name and gender . . .

and make no assumptions. If Dee Walker happens to be a woman and addressed by a job-seeker's letter as "Dear Mr. Walker"—she may be turned off. Personalize your cover letter by using their name on the body of the letter. Other potential problems include misspelled names, incorrect titles, grammatical errors, typographical errors, form letters or ineffective writing, including poor sentence structure.

If an advertisement requests that replies be sent to the director of rehabilitation or to the chief physical therapist, that may be acceptable. However, whenever possible, it is better to identify a person, by calling that department to locate the correct information, because everyone generally prefers to be addressed by his or her own name.

3) Date your cover letter but not your resume. Your resume, as long as it is up-to-date, should not change that much. A date will make it look out-dated when it really is not.

4) Keep your cover letter brief and informal; throw away the parchment paper, typographical gimmicks and the duplicating machine. Make your letter fit on one page; restrain any effort to over-write or over-sell. Never use abbreviations in your cover letter. Use simple direct language. Convey in your closing statement that you would like an appointment with them at their convenience.

5) Be sure to indicate that your resume is enclosed.

6) Regarding format, type the letter on standard size white or ivory paper (8½" x 11"). Leave at least one inch margins on the top, sides, and bottom.

The following sample cover letters should serve as suggestions for you in reaching key people in your marketing campaign. Use them as a guide to develop ideas for your own cover letters, but try to be original.

Sample Cover Letters

To a Target Facility Without a Resume

Mrs. Mary Jackson, P.T.   May 30, 19XX
Director of Rehabilitation
Doctor's Hospital
234 Main Street
Greenwood, Illinois 39482

Dear Ms. Jackson:

I understand that Doctor's Hospital has not yet developed a sports medicine clinic, and in the chance that this subject interests you, I would like to introduce myself.

For the past eight years I have been a sports medicine director for Jackson Hospital in Canton, Ohio. I was instrumental in creating this clinic and it is now staffed with seven full-time staff physical therapists. The clinic now services three high schools, two colleges and is constantly expanding its services.

My family and I are relocating to your area soon and I am interested in continuing my career in sports medicine. My experience in developing a clinic in a community the same size as yours, may be of benefit to you, your facility, and your community.

I would be delighted to meet with you, Ms. Jackson, and explain how I can set up a successful sport medicine clinic within your facility. I will contact you next week to discuss this proposal and to arrange a convenient meeting date.

Thank you for your consideration.

Sincerely,
James White, P.T.

Ms. Janis Baker   July 4, 19XX
69384 Clark Street
Houston, Texas 49382

Dear Janis:

It has been some time since we have talked, and I hope everything is well with you and your family. I often think of the good times we had together in the past.

As you know, I have been working for the last five years as a pediatric therapist at Children's Hospital and enjoy working with children. My husband, Don, has been transferred with his company to your area and we will be moving the end of this month.

I am in the process of preparing a resume and will forward a copy to you. Meanwhile, if you become aware of any pediatric openings in the area, please feel free to refer me to them.

I am looking forward to seeing you soon and am happy to live near you again. Any leads you can give me in my job search will be greatly appreciated.

Thanks for your help.

Sincerely,
Sue Logan

Mr. Walter Hudson, P.T.   January 8, 19XX
President
Hudson and Associates
3493 Main Street
New York, New York 20211

Dear Mr. Hudson:

David Blackson mentioned to me that your company is expanding, and suggested that I should get in touch with you. He spoke highly of you and your company, and I would be delighted to arrange an interview with you.

My experience has been primarily in orthopedics. I have been working at Jones Hospital in New York as a staff physical therapist for the last seven years. We treat mostly orthopedic patients, but also work with neurologic, burns and pediatric patients as well.

I am interested in being a supervisor, but unfortunately my hospital has no positions open. Two co-workers have more seniority than I do, and if an opening should occur, they have priority over me. Therefore, I feel I need to look elsewhere for a management position. David mentioned that you are seeking an orthopedic coordinator, and I feel my background qualifies me for the position.

My resume is enclosed, and I can supply you with more information if needed.

Please get in touch with me to set up an appointment.

Sincerely,
Jack Davidson, P.T.
enclosure: resume

December 5, 19XX

Ms. Linda Jones, O.T.R.
Director of Occupational Therapy
Atlanta Hospital
9847 Peachtree Street
Atlanta, Georgia 30365

Dear Ms. Jones:

Nancy Johnson of Grady Hospital in Atlanta suggested that I contact you concerning opportunities in occupational therapy in Atlanta. As you can see from my enclosed resume, most of my experience in occupational therapy for the last five years has involved young children.

My objective is to relocate to Atlanta this winter, and I am interested in obtaining a position in occupational therapy either in a hospital or school setting, specializing in pediatrics.

Your comments and suggestions regarding any people or situations I should contact would be most appreciated. Perhaps you have an opening in your facility.

I will be coming to Atlanta at the end of January and would like to interview for any pediatric positions available. Please let me know if this will be convenient for you.

Thank you.

Sincerely,
Marsha Johnson, O.T.R.

enclosure: resume

Mr. Jack Smith, P.T.   March 8, 19XX
Therapy Universal Company
5498 Main Street
Jackson, Mississippi 39216

Dear Jack:

It has been quite awhile since we last saw each other, and I hope things are going well with you. I enjoyed the many years we worked together and have often reflected on the memories of the good times we shared.

You may recall that I left the hospital and joined a private practice as a clinic director. The job has been good experience and quite rewarding for me.

We have had a recent reorganization and my position has been eliminated along with a few others. I have begun looking around and thought of you for help since you are always aware of the job market.

Enclosed is my resume. If you hear of any outpatient clinic director positions, I would appreciate your referrals.

Thank you for your help, Jack.

Sincerely,
Mike Jones, P.T.

enclosure: resume

Ms. Diane James, P.T.   July 30, 19XX
Director of Physical Therapy
St. Joseph Hospital
234 Main Street
New York, New York 14607

Dear Ms. James:

I am a graduating senior from Mayo School of
Health Sciences in Rochester, Minnesota. My
graduation date is December 5, 19XX and I am
currently on my third clinical internship at Jones
Hospital in Denver, Colorado.

I am interested in general acute care working with
a wide variety of patients. I would like to hear
from you about any openings for a new graduate
with my qualifications.

I am available to start work right after the examination on December 14, 19XX and would be
very interested in interviewing with you this fall at
your convenience.

Please get in touch with me at home
(507) 398-7777 or by calling me at my dormitory
phone, which is (507) 876-8765.

Ms. James, thank you for any assistance you can
provide.

Sincerely,
Nancy White
enclosure: resume

Mr. Tom Smith   July 30, 19XX
Administrator
Mercy Hospital
234 Main Street
Portland, Maine 39823

Dear Mr. Smith:

As an experienced occupational therapist with nine years of clinical experience, I am interested in your "Chief Occupational Therapist" position. As you will notice on the enclosed resume, I have spent a substantial portion of my occupational therapy career in a supervisory capacity.

My work experience included acute care, rehabilitation, home health care, and pediatrics. I provide direct patient care in a team approach and I enjoy my work. The challenges and rewards of being a chief occupational therapist are what prompted me to contact you.

My salary requirement is in the mid-$30,000s range and I am open to discuss this with you.

I look forward to hearing from you. Please contact me at (202) 874-3982, and if I am not available, please leave a message.

Thank you, Mr. Smith, for your consideration.

Sincerely,
Betty Jones, O.T.R.

enclosure: resume

Ms. Janis Jones, C.P.C.   June 28, 19XX
XYZ Placement Company
2983 Main Street
Sterling, Iowa 39847

Dear Ms. Jones:

I have decided to seek new opportunities in the metropolitan Sterling area. I would like to begin a new job within the next few months as a staff occupational therapist within a hospital.

My major concerns are:

—small to medium facility
—supportive of continuing education
—progressive therapy department with a good team approach
—salary higher than my current $25,000/year

If you know of any positions that would fit these criteria, please get in touch with me. My resume is enclosed.

Thank you for your help, Ms. Jones.

Sincerely,
David Johnson, O.T.R.

enclosure: resume

Mr. John Thompson, O.T.R.   April 3, 19XX
Director of Occupational Therapy
398 Maple Street
Town, California 39847

Dear Mr. Thompson:

I am a junior occupational therapy student at New York University. Your facility is only a few minutes from where I live and I am seeking a part-time position in your department. I have my evenings and weekends free to work.

If you have an assistant or aide position, I would be very interested in working for you. I worked as a nurses' aide for one year at Mercy Hospital. My college grades are excellent and my desire for on-the-job experience is strong.

I am willing to work whatever evening and weekend hours you have available and I would be interested in working in this capacity for the next two years, until I graduate from New York University.

I hope to hear from you soon. My home phone is (203) 988-9876.

Thank you, Mr. Thompson, for your time and assistance.

Sincerely,
Janet Smith

How to Write a Resume that Sells Yourself

"Work consists of whatever a body is obliged to do . . . play consists of whatever a body is not obliged to do," says Tom Sawyer, when contemplating a fence to be painted. In these few words from the 1876 *Adventures of Tom Sawyer,* Samuel Clemens seems to sum up the problems of creating a resume. It is of critical importance and entails a lot of work because you are "obliged to do it."

The resume will not necessarily win you the job, but it can shoot you down if it is poorly done. Some hard-bitten realists among employers say that resumes are often prepared by resume professionals and look pretty much alike. That does not lessen the need for the resume. In fact, it emphasizes the precision with which it should be drafted.

The resume includes relevant facts about you and is a catalog of what you have to offer an employer. It should answer the four "what" questions:

1) What you can do
2) What you have done
3) What you know
4) What kind of job you would like to have

It serves as a focus for your interview and organizes your assets, facts and dates. Most importantly, the resume introduces you to the employer. Even though you may be in *Who's Who In America,* the employer may not know this . . . and your resume will tell the employer this and other crucial factors in a well organized approach.

Your resume should be neither too short or too long. Details can be presented at the interview. Be sure you can deliver any promises made in the resume. Stick to the facts that the prospective employer can relate in regards to the current available position.

Professionally typed resumes are acceptable. However, typesetting and printing is more attractive and may make your resume stand out more than the others.

Misspelled words and uneven margins may not loom in your world, but they are a definite turn-off to an employer.

64

Your challenge is to gain an interview . . . so that you are no longer just so many words on a piece of paper.

After you are interviewed, your resume will be reviewed many times, and a good resume will keep on selling you throughout your interviewing and negotiating process.

The use of an objective will highlight your main desire and tell the employer what you are seeking. Do not use fancy resume paper, slick magazine stock or folders. Stick with white or ivory paper, 8½" x 11", with neat, easy to read, and well organized pages.

Resume Critique

- Omit from your resume any references to:
  Religion
  Color
  Race
  National origin
  Political preferences
  Opinions of previous employers
  Reasons for leaving previous employers
  Previous salaries
  Anticipated salaries

- Do not overcrowd pages (use a second page if necessary, but do not use a third page)

- List your most recent experience first

- Be sure that it is easy to read, clean, and neat

- Omit unnecessary details—keep to the main points

- Do not cite negatives or use overly positive words

- Stay away from professional resume preparers who use fancy paper and are expensive; however, a professional service to typeset your resume is good

- Use matching high-quality white or ivory paper with black ink for your cover letters, resumes, thank-you letters, and envelopes

---

Figure 6: Resume Critique

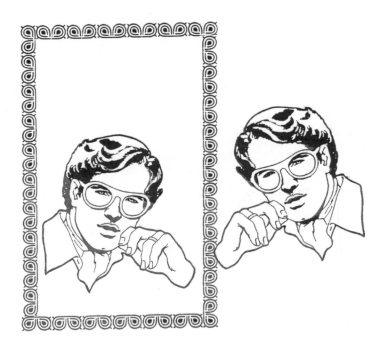

"What do I want to do and who am I?"
Preparing your resume will force you to do a self-evaluation.

Sample Resumes

The following section includes sample resumes. They will aide you in preparing your own.

- The first two are for physical therapists—one for a new graduate and one for an experienced therapist.

- The next two are resumes for occupational therapists—one for a new graduate and one for an experienced therapist.

Use them as a guide in organizing your resume and in developing new ideas.

Suggested Resume Layout for a
New Graduate Physical Therapist

Mary Jones
234 Main Street #49
St. Louis, Missouri 48398
(314) 487-2983 Permanent
(314) 989-3094 School

Career Objective: Seeking a staff physical therapy position in a progressive and rotational clinical setting.

Education: St. Louis University, St. Louis, Missouri
B.S. in Physical Therapy, May, 19XX

Certification: Cardiopulmonary Resuscitation-19XX

Clinical Affiliations:

Senior Year: Barnes Hospital, St. Louis, Missouri—Six weeks of rotation between general rehabilitation, acute care and out-patient services. Emphasis on isokinetic testing and training with equipment such as Biodex and Cybex.

Doctor's Hospital, St. Louis, Missouri—Six weeks of hospital physical therapy procedures with stroke, amputee, and spinal cord injury patients. Conducted the American Back School for chronic pain patients.

Mayo Clinic, Rochester, Minnesota—Six weeks in this nationally recognized facility. Treated unusual disability conditions with innovative treatment techniques. 50% caseload of home-bound clients.

Junior Year: Children's Hospital, Detroit, Michigan—Three weeks in acute care, rehabilitation, and outpatient services. Worked with infants to adolescents in speciality orthopedics, including total shoulder, knee, and hip replacement programs.

Veteran's Administration, Cleveland, Ohio—Three week affiliation with cerebral palsy, mental retardation, and learning disabled children. Emphasis on neurodevelopmental and sensory integration techniques.

Volunteer Experience: 19XX-19XX: Doctor's Hospital, St. Louis, Missouri—Worked in physical and occupational therapy departments as an aide.

Honors and Activities: Dean's List 19XX and 19XX; Student Physical Therapy Association-19XX to present: Treasurer; National Ski Team Patrol: 19XX-present

Licensure: National licensing board exam to be taken on July 11, 19XX

References: St. Louis University Placement Office (314) 558-3847, St. Louis, Missouri; Also Provided Upon Request

Suggested Resume Layout for an Experienced
Physical Therapist

Confidential Resume of:

Joe Hiller, PT
15 Main Street
New York, New York 20293
(212) 398-2039

Career Objective: Seeking a chief therapist position in a medium-sized acute care facility.

Education: Columbia University, New York, New York
M.S. in Physical Therapy-19XX

Boston University, Boston, Massachusetts
B.S. in Physical Therapy-19XX

Licensure: State of New York-I.D.# 39848
State of Maine-I.D.# 309487

Employment:
8-19XX to present: Sinai Hospital, New York, N.Y.
Director of Physical Therapy
Managed rehabilitation department of 3 PT's, 2 aides, 4 assistants, 1 orderly, and two secretaries. Mainly involved with orthopedics, neurologic, and general rehabilitation patients within a 150 bed hospital.

7-19XX to 8-19XX: Mercy Hospital, New York, N.Y.
Staff Physical Therapist
Experience consisted of treatment of general acute-care patients in a 300 bed department with 5 PT's, 3 PT aides, and a secretary. Responsible for developing weekly in-service programs to other medical personnel.

5-19XX to 7-19XX: Denver Hosptial, Denver, CO
Staff Physical Therapist
—This 500 bed acute care hospital is involved with treating joint replacement for knees, hips and spines. Conducted community services in pain management.

Military: United States Air Force - 19XX to 19XX

Professional Organizations: APTA member - 19XX to present: By-Laws Committee Chairman

. . .2

Continuing Education: Dogwood Conference	19XX
Spinal and Extremity Mobilization Seminar	19XX
Pain Management of the Burn Patient	19XX
McKenzie Seminar	19XX
T.M.J. Seminar	19XX
Advance Mobilization Technique	19XX
Laser Seminar	19XX
McKenzie Seminar	19XX
APTA National Conference	19XX
APTA National Conference	19XX
Sports Medicine Seminar	19XX
Stan Paris Seminar	19XX

References: Furnished Upon Request

Suggested Resume Layout for a New Graduate Occupational Therapist

---

Linda Bates
20394 Bay Street
Dayton, Ohio 39847
(513) 983-3984

Career Objective: Seeking an occupational therapy position in a progressive facility which treats primarily psychiatric cases.

Education: Eastern Michigan University, Ypsilanti, Michigan
B.S. in Occupational Therapy, June, 19XX

Certification: Sitting for AOTA national exam on December 5, 19XX, Certified Life Guard-19XX

Clinical Experience:
Senior Year: Children's Hospital, Dayton, Ohio—First six weeks with inpatient boys ranging in ages from 8-14 years old. Diagnoses included: dysthymic depression, attention deficit disorders, substance abuse and schizophrenia. Responsible for weekly patient progress notes. Participated in community outings. Second six weeks with adult psychiatric women ranging from 19-80 years old. Experience with the following diagnoses: character disorders, schizophrenia, and disorders resulting from organic causes. Activities included craft and task groups, group therapy, field trips, and recreational therapy. Represented occupational therapy in weekly team meetings and documented patient progress.

Cleveland Clinic, Cleveland, Ohio—First six weeks worked on the closed head injury team with patients functioning in the Cognitive Levels 3 through 7. Patients ranged from 14-50 years old. Treatment techniques included N.D.T., S.I., Rood and Brunnstrom. Second six weeks worked on the orthopedic team with patients having the following diagnoses: osteoarthritis, hip arthrodesis, total hip replacement, and chronic pain. Performed home evaluations and modifications.

Junior Year worked three weeks each: Psychiatric Hospital of Toledo, Toledo, Ohio (Psychiatric Department); Indiana Hospital, Elkhart, Indiana (Physical Disability Clinic); Suburban Clinic, Lima, Ohio (General Rehabilitation Unit).

Volunteer Experience: 19XX-19XX: Jamestown Hospital, Jamestown, OH. Worked in the occupational therapy department as an assistant.

. . .2

2.

Additional Work Experience: 19XX-19XX: Main Library, Dayton, Ohio; 19XX-19XX: Lifeguard.

Honors and Activities: Dean's List: 19XX and 19XX; Student Occupational Therapy Association: 19XX to Present: President; *Who's Who Among Students in American Colleges and Universities*-19XX.

References: Eastern Michigan University Placement Office (313) 487-0275, Ypsilanti, Michigan; Also Provided Upon Request

Suggested Resume Layout for an Experienced
Occupational Therapist

David Jones, O.T.R.
6409 Brown Street
Columbus, Ohio 49827
(614) 934-3948

Career Objective: Seeking a staff occupational therapy position in an acute care setting.

Education: College of St. Catherine, St. Paul, Minnesota
B.S. in Occupational Therapy, June, 19XX

Certification: American Occupational Therapy Association-Registration #029382

Employment:

8-19XX to present: Ohio State School, Columbus, Ohio
Staff occupational therapist
Evaluated and treated severely mentally and physically handicapped children and adults using development techniques and activities of daily living.

8-19XX to 8-19XX: Dayton Children's Training Center, Dayton, Ohio
Staff occupational therapist
Worked with developmentally delayed children from 0-3 years old. Treatment plans included gross and fine motor activities, communication skills, and self-care activities.

3-19XX to 7-19XX: University Hospital, Cleveland, Ohio
Staff occupational therapist
Treated 50 mentally ill adults using group activities, crafts, and created adaptive splinting in evaluating and treatment of these patients.

9-19XX to 2-19XX: Springfield School, Springfield, Ohio
Staff occupational therapist
Worked in a public school with mentally retarded, physically handicapped and learning disabled students. Children were primarily involved in progressive therapy techniques geared to independent living.

7-19XX to 8-19XX: Rehabilitation Institute of Ohio, Columbus, Ohio
Staff occupational therapist
Rotated at the center and local hospitals with adults and children who were physically handicapped, emotionally disturbed, or mentally retarded 35-40 patients. Assisted O.T. Director with community awareness services.   ...2

2.

Professional Organizations: AOTA member-19XX to present

Continuing Education: National AOTA Conference 19XX, 19XX; Pain Management Seminar-19XX; Rehabilitation of the Child-19XX; NDT Workshop-19XX; Splinting Workshop-19XX

References: Furnished upon request.

CHAPTER 4
The Interview

- Doing Your Homework
- Dressing to Get the Job
- Traveling
- Arriving on Time
- The Waiting Room
- The First Interview Contact
- Filling Out Application Forms
- The Interview Conversation
- Meals During Interviews
- Positives and Negatives of Job Interviews
- Interview Questions
- Tricky Questions You Should Be Able to Answer
- Telephone Manners and Test
- Post Interview Etiquette
  1. Thank You Letter After a Direct Interview
  2. Thank You Letter Declining an Offer

CHAPTER 4
The Interview

On the other side of the employment looking glass sits the employer, who might advise applicants to not try to pretend to be someone else or to say what you think the employer wants to hear. Most employers can spot a phony and they have had plenty of experience. So be yourself!

Perhaps it will put you at ease to know that "interview" comes from the French word *intervoir,* meaning "visit each other." Now that sounds tame enough, doesn't it? Your objective is to get a job offer; the interviewer's objective is to identify the best candidate for the job. Remember, too, that your visit always involves a third party—a hospital, organization, clinic or agency—which completes the interview triangle. This silent third party, which determines responsibilities for quality care and costs of operation, impacts greatly on candidate selection.

You need to plan your interview just as you would study for a test, realizing that it is a structured conversation with two parts—talking and listening. Both parts are important in helping you demonstrate composure and in controlling the situation.

Whether you are a new graduate or an experienced therapist, you are bound to be nervous, but the interviewer does not need to know that. You should appear eager, but not too eager. Your emotions are in conflict, bubbling and boiling, but in the words of an ubiquitous TV commercial, "Never let them see you sweat." Those destined for interview success project a natural, confident, pleasant and knowledgeable manner. You must not look uneasy or appear to "dig your toe in the carpet" if asked questions you can not answer.

If you arrive at the interview mentally prepared for success, you will have an edge over the competition. You might even enjoy the interview and decide it was a rewarding experience.

The most common interview with a physical therapist or occupational therapist will be done by:

1) The personnel or human resources department representative
2) The rehabilitation manager
3) Other management personnel

To appear successful in any interview situation, you are encouraged to do some work and follow certain rules. If you do, you will not appear timid or unsure of yourself.

As we will now proceed to review the interview steps from the initial step of doing your homework and proceeding in to the initial interview, please refer periodically to Figure 9—Positives and Negatives in Job Interviews.

Doing Your Homework

You should know the types of patient health services provided by your prospective employer. You do not have to know every detail in the annual report, but it helps to know some of the background and of the current operations of the facility. If it has won awards, be familiar with them. Perhaps services are being expanded or there is a building project underway.

Libraries often can help you with this type of information through their local newspapers, annual reports, and periodical sections. In addition, literature can usually be obtained directly from the facility, prior to the interview.

Occasionally, employers will ask what you know about the hospital or clinic. If the organization has earned a reputation for a certain specialty, you would do well to indicate that you are aware of the fact. Perhaps the interviewer will mention a specific problem; you then can explain how you could be part of the solution.

If you understand the concerns of the employer, you will be in a better position to show how you can help. Be prepared to demonstrate a broad knowledge of the health care industry. This includes a passing acquaintance with the components of health care delivery, which include:

1) public sector
2) private sector
3) ambulatory care
4) health maintenance organizations/preferred provider organizations
5) home health care agencies

(See Figures 7 and 8)

Also take a look at how health care services are being financed. Someone once said, "A fellow who can see both sides of a question equally obviously doesn't have anything invested in it." That is not true of your prospective employer; for he or she has a definite investment and takes the question of payment seriously. The methods of financing health care services are:

1) public and private plans
2) prospective plans
3) national health insurance

A good source of information on institutions, organizations, and agencies in the health care field is *The American Hospital Association Guide to the Health Care Field,* published by the American Hospital Association. This guide provides a variety of information about each hospital, including the administrator's name; various approvals; selected services and facilities; relationship to the multihospital system; classification by control; service; average length of stay; and selected statistical data from AHA.

Other reference sources can be found in public libraries, college and university libraries; trade institute/industry libraries; newspapers—local, regional, national; directories; information retrieval services; and trade journals. (See Appendix for a listing of references and resources.)

Figure 7: **Physical Therapists Practice Settings**

Percent employed by work setting, 1986

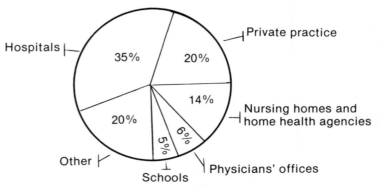

Source: *Occupational Outlook Handbook*
Bureau of Labor Statistics
U.S. Department of Labor
April '88, Bulletin 2300; page 145

Figure 8: **Types of Patients Occupational Therapists Service**

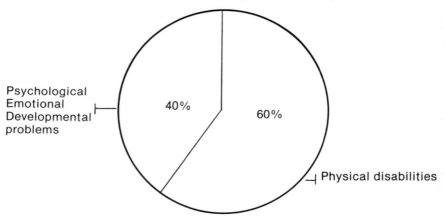

Source: *Occupational Outlook Handbook*
Bureau of Labor Statistics
U.S. Department of Labor
April '88, Bulletin 2300; page 138

Dressing to Get the Job

In order to gain the best response, dress appropriately. If you neglect your appearance, employers may assume that you have poor self-image. You are judged by your physical characteristics and personality, so take a tip from the words of an old Sunday school song and "let your light shine through."

Even though the physical therapy or rehabilitation department is a relaxed environment where therapists dress casually, this does not mean casual dress is expected at the job interview. You should dress as a professional person—neatly and well groomed. A man should wear a conservative blue or black suit, a long sleeved white shirt with a matching tie and black polished shoes. A woman should wear a conservative suit or dress in navy, tan or gray. V-necks, high hemlines and flashy jewelry are inappropriate. Also avoid carrying large briefcases and purses, heavy perfume and excessive makeup.

You are not applying for a job on TV's ever-popular M.A.S.H. unit, where all forms of attire were fictionally allowed; you are seeking employment in the real world of dress codes. In this world, employers usually have conservative requirements regarding the clothing their employees wear.

Traveling

Whether your interview is across town or across the country, ask for directions to the interview site, and include enough details to help you find your destination. Write down and take along the telephone number where you are expected for the interview. Some places are obscure even in the best of times. But driving too fast in heavy traffic, while looking for unfamiliar street signs, will not lower your blood pressure on your interview day. So plan enough time for the trip. Making a dry-run a few days prior to the interview will avoid you getting late or being nervous on your scheduled interview day.

Make sure you have any necessary maps in your car and study your route in advance. Take along plenty of change for metered parking and phone calls. You have prepared well, and as extra insurance, arrive in a car that is clean and neat. You may be asked to take someone at the interview site to another location.

Arrive on Time

Be on time. Interviewers place high value on the punctuality of your arrival. If you reach their parking lot early, sit and listen to the radio . . . it will relax you. Getting to the receptionist's desk more than five or ten minutes early can put unwelcomed pressure on the interviewer.

Unavoidably, if you are arriving late, stop and call ahead and let the secretary know that you may be a few minutes late. You show courtesy by calling ahead and you also may avoid having your interview cancelled. There is no excuse for being late for an interview. It leaves the impression that you are neither time conscious nor considerate.

Avoid the misfortune of a bad first impression by leaving for your interview at least one hour early, in case you get hung up in traffic. Why drive white-knuckled and arrive at one of the most important meetings of your life disheveled and breathless? Planning ahead helps. Try not to squeeze in the interview on a day already packed with other commitments. If possible, choose a day that promises to have the time you need to invest in your future. It will improve your chances of not getting nervous and allow you to display your best side.

If the interviewer asks, "Did you have any trouble finding us?" the best answer is always, "No." As a therapist responsible for mapping a patient care program, you do not want a prospective employer to believe that you cannot find your way around the block. Why give the interviewer the impression that you received inadequate directions, even if you did? Part of your training as a professional is to check things out for yourself.

The Waiting Room

When Longfellow said "All things come round to him who will but wait," he probably had not spent too much time in waiting rooms. There is truth in what he said, but perhaps little understanding of what one can or cannot do while waiting for an interview. For example, in the late 1940s, a certain young therapist, while sitting in a psychiatric waiting room with patients, smoked a cigarette, and finding no receptacle, dunked the ashes into his pants' cuff. As the patients mimicked his behavior, he became concerned that he might not be recognized as a therapist. Eventually he was properly identified and rescued by Dr. Yoder, who at that time headed Ypsilanti State Hospital in Michigan.

A few tips on handling the waiting room trial can help. Try to be comfortable but do not slouch, and stay within the reception area. When you are called to "be on stage," make sure you are not in the cafeteria getting coffee. Remember, interviewing may not be fair, but you are the one at a disadvantage.

The interview may not be relaxing to you, but try not to let any annoyance show. Everyone wants to know what to do with things they may bring to the interview . . . an outer coat, umbrella, hat and gloves. Leave them in the reception room.

Be polite to everyone from the parking attendant to the secretary. At the same time, do not get too familiar with the receptionist or the secretaries; your conversation can be taken the wrong way and may be misrepresented to their superior.

While waiting you can read about the organization in the brochures, annual reports and advertising pieces that are usually displayed in the waiting room. Or you may want to take the time to review your resume. Do not smoke, chew gum or accept candy, if offered. You may take a cup of coffee or tea, if asked by someone. Your waiting capability has to be high because it will be tested many times as a job applicant.

If you are kept too long in the waiting room, you must

consider other appointments. If you know you are going to be late, phone ahead and reschedule your next meeting. Ask the receptionist if there is a pay phone nearby where you can make a call. Do not use the office phone unless it is an emergency situation.

First Interview Contact

If the interviewer calls you by your first name, do not assume you should do the same. It is safer to use "Mr., Miss or Ms.," but do not make an issue of it by asking. Using "Miss or Ms." is safe, because she can take the initiative on correcting you.

Your handshake should be neither limp nor bone-crushing. Sit down only when invited to do so. Pay attention to what is happening and focus on the person interviewing you. Remember to smile and nod your head, but not constantly. Listen and look interested in what the interviewer is saying. Give him or her the satisfaction of feeling important . . . because it is the truth. Do not be like a youngster in an autograph-seeking frenzy at the ballpark, who runs up to a player he does not recognize and says: "Are you anybody?"

Filling Out Application Forms

Many employers will have you fill out an application as a document for their files and as a protective measure. Unlike a resume, an application carries your signature and has the force of law behind it.

It is a good idea to prepare an application form and carry it with you to the interview (see Figure 9: Application Form). This can be used as a crib sheet for names, phone numbers, dates, etc., at your actual interview site and will show preparation and good planning.

Be neat and answer all questions truthfully. The information can be checked and, if it is false in any part, can cost you the chance of being hired. If the truth is revealed after you have the job, you can still be fired. The information regarding your education, training and experience as a therapist should be a matter of verifiable facts.

Figure 9: **Application Form**

Name _____ Soc. Security #_____

Address _____

City _____ State _____ Zip _____

Phone ( ) _____

College Degree   Bachelors _____ Year _____

                   Master _____ Year _____

If Emergency, Contact: Name _____ Phone _____

                        Address _____

Employment History—List last facility first

1. Name _____   Type of Facility _____
   Address _____   City _____ State ____
   Job Title _____   Dates of Employment _____

2. Name _____   Type of Facility _____
   Address _____   City _____ State ____
   Job Title _____   Dates of Employment _____

3. Name _____   Type of Facility _____
   Address _____   City _____ State ____
   Job Title _____   Dates of Employment _____

List of Professional References

       Name   Address   Phone

1. _____

2. _____

3. _____

Professional Licenses

_____ expiration date _____

_____ expiration date _____

Professional Organization and Associations

_____

_____

_____

The Interview Conversation

Reflecting on one's ability to talk rather than listen, Thomas Edison said, "God invented the talking machine. I only invented the first one that can shut off." His observation should be taken as a warning to job seekers—you are not expected to talk all the time.

At the interview, listen intently and take a moment to think over your replies. Demonstrate as much knowledge as possible about research in physical or occupational therapy, but do not bluff your way through such questions. Prospective employers appreciate honesty; tell them what you know.

Tell the truth without being defensive; admit it when you are unfamiliar with something. You have credentials and you should be proud of them. Speak slowly and clearly with a matter-of-fact sincerity, and avoid using "ah," "you know," "yeah," or other verbal slips. Be patient and do not interrupt; you will get your turn in the conversation.

You should never say negative things about present or past employers; show that you are capable and loyal. Also, do not reveal any confidential information from any previous employer.

Since the interview is a conversation, you should listen at least 51% of the time. Do not monopolize the conversation; it is not up to you to control the situation. Let the employers control the interview.

Interviews often are not limited to your area of expertise, so be prepared to show a diversity of knowledge on other subjects. Will Rogers once said: "There's nothing so stupid as the educated man if you get off the subject he's educated in."

Meals During Interviews

You may be invited to lunch as a step in the interview process. Many high level administrative therapy positions include a lunch or dinner interview. If you have been invited,

Figure 10: **Positives and Negatives of Job Interviews**

Positives

1. Knows something about the company
2. Has a specific job or jobs in mind
3. Has reviewed job qualifications
4. Is prepared to answer broad questions
5. Is self-confident, but not egotistical
6. Is straight forward and honest
7. Has good conversational ability
8. Has good scholastic ability
9. Has good work history
10. Has good appearance
11. Asks good questions
12. Is a good listener
13. Projects responsibility
14. Will travel if asked
15. Is not a job hopper
16. Shows ambition and initiative
17. Displays empathy on patient care quality
18. Has a good personality
19. Is self motivated
20. Takes resume to interview

Negatives

1. Has untidy appearance (i.e., shoes unshined, hair not groomed, dressed incorrectly, fingernails dirty, too much makeup)
2. Talks excessively
3. Criticizes previous employer
4. Overstresses money
5. Will not consider relocation
6. Is late for interview
7. Answers too briefly, talks too fast
8. Lacks enthusiasm
9. Has a weak handshake
10. No eye contact
11. Chews gum
12. Sloppy in completing application blank
13. Smokes during interview
14. Is not honest
15. Has poor grammar, poise, diction
16. Is not prepared for the interview
17. Lacks tact, maturity, courtesy
18. Slouches, fidgets, looks at floor instead of interviewer
19. Puts hand over mouth when talking or uses hands excessively
20. Acts nervous or shaky

accept the invitation. You will find yourself being observed by several people. This is another measure used to predict your performance.

Order foods which will not be sloppy or hard to manage. If asked about a drink, ask for a soft drink or mineral water. You do not want to be impaired at this important time in the interview, nor do you want to come across as a drinker. If you are not sure what to order for an entree, take your cue from others with you. If they are all ordering a sandwich or salad, you do not want them to wait for your well-done steak to be cooked. Pick something easy and take small bites so you are prepared to answer questions.

Avoid smoking, and if you are on a diet, keep quiet about it. The subject has been talked to death, and no one wants to hear about it over a business lunch.

Social graces and table manners come together with what your mother always taught you, so remember to be polite and be at your best. When you say goodbye, do remember to thank the interviewer.

Interview Questions

There are several questions you need to have answered in order to understand what the job is really about. They may be covered by the interviewer in your conversation (also see page 114 -Figure 13: Outline of Employee Concerns). The following questions must be answered; if not, ask them before the interview is terminated. *Ask them selectively* and only *when appropriate* to the conversation.

1) What is the size of the facility? How many beds are there and what is your current occupancy? If it is a 450-bed facility, does this include your 30-bed rehabilitation floor? If it is a multi-facility operation, how many clinics or sites are there and where are the locations?

2) Is your organization profit or non-profit? How is it funded?

3) What is the daily average caseload per staff therapist on each shift? What is the patient to therapist ratio?

4) How many therapists are employed in the depart-

ment? How many physical therapists, occupational therapists, aides, and assistants are there? Are these employees full-time or part-time?

5) What type of patients do you treat (i.e., orthopedic, neurologic, general rehabilitation, psychiatric)? In what areas do you specialize?

6) What treatment procedures are being used (electrical stimulation, pain suppressors, equipment and set-ups, etc.)?

7) Does your rehabilitation department include physical therapy, occupational therapy, speech therapy, and audiology? Or are these separate departments? Where are these departments located?

8) At what facility will I be placed and for how long? Will I have the opportunity to rotate and learn at your other locations?

9) Can I visit the actual office where I will be working?

10) May I see your job description?

11) Is this a staff or supervisory position?

12) What are the major responsibilities of the job?

13) Why is this position available?

14) Who worked here before and for how long? Why did this person leave?

15) How long has this position been open?

16) What are the most common reasons for turnover in this organization?

17) What are the termination policies?

18) To whom do I report?

19) If considering relocation, what costs are paid for? What is the size of the town? What is the standard of living?

20) What is the methodology used to evaluate an employee?

21) What is the work schedule? How often is it revised?

22) Do you have a probationary period and if so for how long?

23) What types of benefits are available? When do they go into effect? What is your vacation policy? What types of health insurance (including dental and vision) are offered and who pays? Do you provide malpractice coverage? Is

there a budget for continuing education and tuition reimbursement? Is there profit sharing? Is there a sign-on bonus? Are there any other benefits?

24) Is my starting date acceptable to you? Will previous vacation plans be allowed?

25) What is the annual salary of this position? Are there yearly increases or cost of living allowances? (Do not discuss salary at the beginning—focus on the job.)

Tricky Questions You Should Be Able to Answer

You will be asked many questions during your interview and some may be questions you never expected to be asked. Here are some questions which will help you to be prepared prior to your interview:

1) *What do you think of your previous employer?* The best advice for this is to stay neutral. Neither say anything overly positive or negative. Criticizing your former employer will make you appear as a complainer. Try to portray your experiences in terms of learning from beneficial situations. For example, "The new rehab floor had a very heavy volume of patients, which gave me good experience in treating many rehab patients."

2) *Tell me about yourself.* Give a brief summary of your career beginning with your education and through your work experiences. Add one or two accomplishments along the way and be positive. Do not talk over five minutes and be prepared to speak about your skills and why you are suited for the job opening.

3) *Why did you leave your previous job?* Work out rational reasons for your job moves. Give positive reasons why you changed jobs, such as advancement opportunities, salary increases, challenges, responsibilities, or other reasons. Do not use reasons such as: you did not get along with your co-workers or boss; you did not like certain changes; you were passed over for a raise; you had too many patients and too much pressure; you did not like rehabilitation patients; you had too much work; you had too much overtime and they were short of staff all the time; you had

bad health; you had personal problems; you had too many arguments; or other negative stories.

4) *Can you work under pressure?* Indicate that you are used to working under pressure and ask, "How much and what kind of pressure is involved with this job?"

5) *What salary do you expect?* Try to stress that the opportunities and experiences are more important to you than the salary. Ask back, "What is your salary range?" You should tell the interviewer your present salary if asked.

6) *In your opinion, what are your strengths and weaknesses?* Emphasize your strengths and assets as they relate to the desired position. As to your weaknesses, do not criticize yourself too much, but say, for example, "I get impatient sometimes because I like to get things done quickly; but I'm better at controlling my impatience and dealing with the situation at hand."

7) *What do you know about our company?* This question will reveal your homework. By indicating your knowledge of the facility, you will display your intelligence and interest. A complete lack of knowledge shows that you did not take the time to prepare for this interview.

8) *Describe your management style.* This is a leadership question and should be answered carefully. Stress how well you handle the delegation of duties while maintaining quality control. Discuss leadership styles and examples of your management. Mention that you treat people well and how well you motivate them as loyal employees. Relate actual examples that demonstrate management traits.

9) *Do you prefer to work in small, medium, or large facilities?* Ask for clarification of numbers of employees or patients. Relate this to the interview in process and answer accordingly. (If you are prepared, you should know the vital statistics.)

10) *What types of patients do you prefer to treat?* This question will show your varied interests. If the facility does not service the patient load you indicate, you will not fit their needs and probably will not get the job. However, by indicating flexibility and a wide range of interests, you will become a more suitable candidate.

11) *How long have you been looking for a job?* If you have been searching over 6 months or longer, you should mention if you have been doing any consulting or part-time work. Relate volunteer or other human service work. If you are still employed, explain that you keep your eyes open for better opportunities, and that this job particularly appealed to you because of (cite example).

12) *Why are you interested in changing jobs?* You can say that you are seeking greater opportunities, increased personal or professional growth, or new challenges. If it is because of a change in location, say so. Do not stress money as the primary motive in changing jobs.

13) *Do you like to travel?* If you do not know how much travel is involved, ask the interviewer for your job related travel requirements. Then decide if this matches your needs.

14) *Are you considering any other positions at this time?* You do not need to reveal the names of other facilities or employers, if there are any. This is confidential information. You may want to indicate that you are considering a "few" positions, but do not give the impression that you are interviewing everywhere.

Telephone Manners

The first few seconds of a phone call are critical because you are making your first impression. Your rate of speech should match that of the person to whom you are talking. Your voice should sound warm, friendly, and professional. Do not transmit impatience or frustration as this will cause a negative reaction from the interviewer and decrease your chances for a job.

If you have an answering machine, let the machine pick up the calls instead of the family. Your recorded message should be friendly, businesslike, clear, and easy to understand, and never cute or musical. Identify yourself and simply ask the caller to leave his or her name, telephone number, time of the call, and a brief message.

When placing a business call, be sure you have the correct name and telephone number. Make your calls within reasonable business hours—9:00 a.m. to 5:00 p.m.—unless otherwise specified by the party you are calling.

As soon as your call is answered, identify yourself, and the name of your organization. Give your name briefly and explicitly as possible in a calm, clear voice. "This is Mary Johnson of Mercy Hospital in Detroit. May I please speak to David Smith?"

If the person answering says, "Mr. Smith is busy with a patient now," simply leave your complete name, the name of your organization, and the phone number. Thank the person and say goodbye, as you would in face-to-face conversation. If you decide to omit the name of your facility, indicate when you can be reached at home and leave your home phone number. Do not slam down or drop the phone into the receiver; the person at the other end may still have the phone close to his or her ear and the sudden noise could be annoying as well as rude. (See Appendix in Phone Log.)

Telephone Manners Test

Here are some questions to test your telephone manners. The more you answer "yes" to it, the better your telephone manners.

	Yes	No
1) Do you call collect to an employer by permission only?	☐	☐
2) Do you make business calls within the normal business hours of 9:00 a.m. to 5:00 p.m. (unless instructed otherwise)?	☐	☐
3) Do you avoid making personal calls at work unless on your lunch break or at a pay phone?	☐	☐
4) Do you make sure your conversation is as brief as possible, without appearing too short?	☐	☐
5) Do you avoid dragging out the conversation?	☐	☐
6) Do you keep a pen and paper handy next to the phone?	☐	☐
7) Do you set up an interview/appointment within a reasonable period of time (a couple of weeks)?	☐	☐

Post-Interview Etiquette

Telephone manners are fairly easy to master with practice and patience, while writing skills may be a little more troublesome. In either case, the ability to communicate is important. Weak written communication skills can be improved with a good basic writer's manual.

Writing thank-you notes after the interview is a part of the post-interview etiquette. Being courteous is just as important as the interview. You may not work at the facility you just interviewed with; however you may decide two years later that you want to go back and talk with them.

Thank the person for taking the time spent with you and perhaps add a kind comment or two about the person or the company. The thank-you note should be typed and should contain only three or four paragraphs.

The following pages are examples of thank-you notes that should be written within 48 hours of the interview:

1) Sample thank-you letter after a direct interview
2) Sample thank-you letter declining an offer

Also, do not forget to write to your friends or business contacts to thank them for their help and notifying them of your new position.

Thank-You Letter After a Direct Interview

David Jones, P.T.
139 Bell Road
Jackson, Florida 43092
(914) 398-3984

March 9, 19XX

Ms. Kate Johnson, P.T., M.P.H.
Director of Rehabilitation
Jones Hospital
948 E. Main Street
Jackson, Florida 39823

Dear Ms. Johnson:

It was a pleasure to meet you and your staff. I enjoyed discussing your needs for a qualified physical therapist.

As you may recall, my experience in pediatrics is extensive and would tie in well with your plans for the pediatric floor, as well as your need for an experienced pediatric physical therapist.

Thank you for your time and interest, and the tour of your department. I would welcome hearing from you soon. The opportunity to work for you is quite appealing to me.

Sincerely,

David Jones, P.T.

Mary Smith, O.T.R.
167 Main Street
Denver, Colorado 49834

July 17, 19XX

Mr. Tom Jones, O.T.R.
Director of Occupational Therapy
Mercy Hospital
578 Pine Street
Rivertown, Colorado 29832

Dear Mr. Jones:

Thank you very much for the interview last Monday, July 15, 19XX. I appreciate the opportunity to meet you and your rehabilitation staff.

I want to let you know that I have just accepted another job offer locally and will start work soon. Your position was high on my list of potential choices and it was difficult for me to decide.

Again, Mr. Jones, thank you for all your time and interest.

Sincerely,

Mary Jones, O.T.R.

CHAPTER 5
Through the Employer's Eyes

- Strategies of Staffing: Retention and Recruitment
  1. Encourage Professional and Career Advancement
  2. Form an Alliance with the Personnel or Human Resources Department
  3. Use Replacement Planning and Forecasting Future Staffing Needs
  4. Provide Alternative Work Schedules Options
  5. Promote or Transfer Internally
  6. Create a Job Description
  7. Organize an Effective Advertising Campaign
  8. Offer Competitive Salaries and Benefits
  9. Commit to Educational Programs
  10. Award Scholarships and/or Stipends to Students
  11. Make Professional Presentations and Publish Articles
  12. Allow Senior Staff Members to Teach
  13. Sponsor Student Clinical Education Programs
  14. Develop Work-Study Programs
  15. Recruit Informally by Word-of-Mouth
  16. Offer Interview and Relocation Expenses Plus Sign-On Bonuses
  17. Provide Housing for a Specified Time
  18. Attend Local Career Fairs and Sponsor Open Houses
  19. Use Professional Recruiting Agencies
  20. Recruit Internationally
- Outline of Employee Concerns
- Contracting Companies: A Staffing Alternative
- Employing Physical and Occupational Therapy Assistants

CHAPTER 5
Through the Employer's Eyes

Do you think the day will ever come when therapists will compete one on one with robots for careers in patient care? So far, it appears that employers at health care facilities dismiss the notion of artificial intelligence replacing human reasoning in treating patients. Still, if hospital administrators and clinic directors are not rushing out to buy robots, then how are they trying to solve their staffing needs?

It would be wise to look at hiring from the viewpoint of the employer. His or her basic objective is probably much the same as the employees—to provide quality patient care. While maintaining high standards of quality employers need to provide environments conductive to patient care. In this low supply, high demand area of therapists, many times the employer does not think about the hiring process until an employee slaps a resignation letter on their desk.

Managers with insufficient personnel seek help in today's recruitment arena, using strategies that were unheard of years ago. They are forced to predict turnover and maintain active recruitment of new graduates. Competition for therapists keeps increasing as the supply decreases.

Employers can not wait for the market to improve; their facilities will lose patient referrals and money if they wait. This poses a real threat to the growth of the organization. A lack of therapists results in long waited periods for patient treatment—a reputation no institution can afford. Most family doctors are quick to sense if therapists are not able to take all the patient referrals and can not provide services. When this happens, physicians often begin making referrals to other facilities. Here are some possible strategies for staffing, including retention and recruiting.

Strategies of Staffing: Retention and Recruitment

1. *Encourage professional and career advancement* with your staff by allotting time to get to know your staff and understanding their interests and needs. The National Institute of Business Management in New York, New York, reports the following management practices:

• *Encourage open communications* through frequent meetings. About 70% of all performance problems come from employees not knowing what is expected of them. This communication gap leaves employees in the dark. Weekly meetings to clarify new developments and to discuss goals create a stable and controlled environment.

• *Encourage contributions.* Allow your staff to know that you value contributions and that you encourage involvement. This gives your employees a feeling of ownership and openness, and tells them their ideas mean value to the company.

• *Provide feedback by performance reviews.* By doing informal periodic performance reviews, you can talk to your employees about their work. Try to cite specific examples rather than randomly discussing their performance. For example, "In the future, always remember to record in the progress notes Mr. Smith's treatment plan and home instructions." You stand a better chance of getting a favorable response if you reward positive behavior and correct negative behavior in a constructive, caring manner.

• *Offer job rotation.* Many therapists enjoy rotating through different areas they would like to explore. For example, offer to rotate staff therapist Mary Jones through the rehabilitation unit, the out-patient clinic and the home care program. This opens her options, makes her feel needed, and eventually she may want to specialize in just one area.

• *Offer new responsibilities.* Give employees new areas of responsibilities and a chance to assume a leadership role. This will give the employees a chance to prove what they can do. For example, ask your therapists if anyone would like to develop a research project. Or you may ask for volunteers for problem-solving task forces. Compliment your staff for their initiative in accepting the new responsibility or perhaps reward them.

2. Managers of therapy departments should form an *alliance with the personnel or human resources department.* This "partnership" can accomplish a number of objectives:

• It helps to keep the search for therapists a high priority. Otherwise, personnel departments tend to be distracted by the rapid turnover in the departments of nursing, housekeeping, and dietary. In maintaining high priority in recruiting therapists, it may be necessary to assign a full-time personnel representative in this recruiting function or hire another full-time staff recruiter.

• It can focus attention on recruitment methods other than advertising, which personnel departments tend to rely on. Repeated advertisements for therapists may raise the unwarranted suspicion that something unfavorable is causing the turnover.

• It can help the personnel department better understand the duties of physical and occupational therapists, so they can take a more active role in recruiting for these positions. The organizational layout and interactions of other allied health professionals is also better clarified. (See Figure 11: Traditional Organizational Diagram—Rehabilitation Department, and Figure 12: Modern Rehabilitation Department—Patient and Family Centered Model.) It helps if therapy managers provide tours of their departments to the personnel staff, along with demonstrations of patient care duties and introduction to their staff.

• It enables the therapy managers and staff to learn new labor laws, the institution's hiring requirements, and employee benefits.

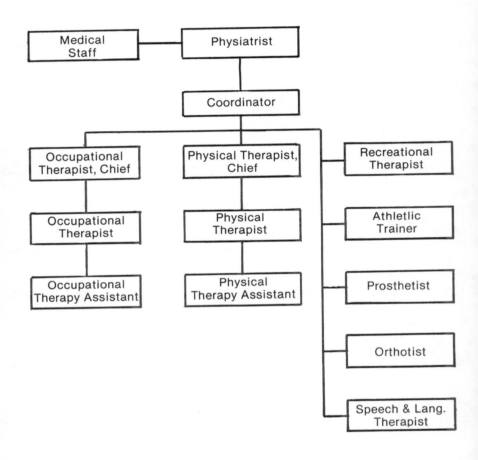

Figure 11: **Traditional Organizational Layout—
Rehabilitation Department**

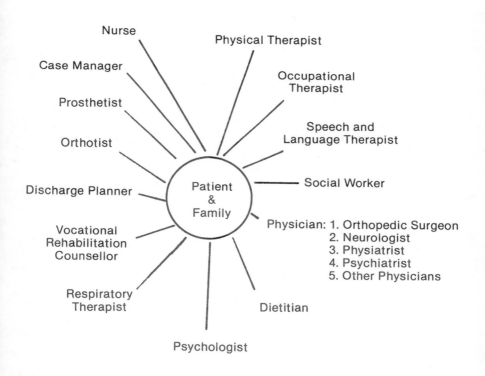

Figure 12: **Modern Rehabilitation Department—
Patient and Family Centered Model**

Experienced managers believe that cooperation and communications between therapy and personnel benefits both departments, and helps give the impression of a well organized facility to applicants for therapy positions. As part of the hiring process, managers know that they must present a consistent, progressive, and positive image to candidates. Towards that end, successful managers maintain professional visibility by keeping their people aware of current issues and practices. Obviously, highly motivated therapists are attracted to dynamic departments.

3. Another defense against personnel shortages continues to be the tactic of *using replacement planning* (otherwise known as "attriting the position"), and *forecasting future staffing needs*. Replacement is when a therapist is hired even though there is no vacant position in the organization. To justify this maneuver, employers reason that a position will eventually open up, due to expected attrition or an increase in the number of patients. Employers can also use forecasting future staffing needs, from one to ten years in advance, and hire as needed. Managers try to ensure they have the right number of people, placed at the right locations and at the right time, doing the tasks that are economically the most useful. This practice attempts to challenge the vicissitudes of the future and the vagaries of the past with varying amounts of success, but still it continues. Prediction of staffing needs, unpredictable at best, seem to have a better success rate when made by health care providers who have been around long enough to have a "track record."

4. *Providing alternative work schedules options by including part-time employment, job sharing, and flexible scheduling,* assists as an effective recruitment program. This can be practical from many standpoints and will appeal to women and those desiring to further their education. According to Pamela Hayes in *Clinical Management* (1989, No. 2), employers need to try harder to meet the personal needs of workers, particularly women with children. Many times duties can be divided among personnel already on staff.

Hayes further explains the alternative work schedule options in job sharing and flexible scheduling as:

A. *Compressed Workweek:* Full time work scheduled in less than five days a week.

B. *Flextime:* Permits flexible starting and quitting times but requires a standard number of hours within a given time period.

C. *Five to Four Nine-Hour Days:* Work five nine-hour days the first week, four nine-hour days the next week, and have the tenth day off.

D. *Four-Day Workweek:* Work four ten-hour days per week.

E. *Job Sharing:* Two therapists sharing the workload of one full-time position, with salary and benefits prorated or negotiated.

F. *Permanent Part-Time:* Work less than full-time with all rights available to full-time employees.

5. In recruitment, many employers believe what Judy Garland said at the end of *The Wizard of Oz:* "Oh, Auntie Em, there's no place like home!" Health care managers will often look "around the house" giving present employees the first chance for *promotion or transfer internally.* According to employers, recruiting candidates from inside the organization has the following benefits:

• encourages employees to feel more secure; builds positive attitudes; and provides goals to which they can attain.

• offers seniority to employees and encourages them to remain with the organization.

• enables retention of experienced employees who are familiar with the organization and its methods of operation. Hiring from the outside always involves a period of organization and training in both policies and procedure, along with additional expenses.

6. Once the necessity of a position has been determined, the employer usually lists applicant qualifications, such as technical skills, special education, people skills, detail ability,

and creativity. Out of this analysis the employer *creates a job description*—the cornerstone of the agreement between the employer and the new employee. It establishes a written reference guide to:

- Outline the duties of the position
- Summarize all work assignments
- Clarify which personnel are assigned to specific duties
- Serve as a basis of employee evaluation
- Establish a positive rapport between the employee and supervisor
- Describe the chain of command

Most job descriptions include to whom to report, gives a broad summary statement of the position, defines the minimum requirements, and provides a detailed explanation of duties. Since this represents an agreement between the applicant and the employer, there should be a place for both the employee and employer to sign the job description.

The following pages provide a sample job description for a director of physical therapy.

Sample Job Description

Main Hospital
Plainsville, New York

JOB DESCRIPTION

Classification:	Reports to:	Department:
Physical Therapy Director:	Administrator:	Physical Therapy Approved by:
Effective Date: June 1, 19XX	Replaces Job Description Dated: 19XX	

I. General Summary: The Director of Physical Therapy assumes responsibility for the administrative functions of the physical therapy department. Also, the director performs patient services, and supervises and coordinates activities in the physical therapy program.
The Assistant Director of Physical Therapy will have the same responsibilities as the Director, assume responsibility when the Director is absent and assist the Director when requested.

II. Minimum Requirements: A Bachelor of Science Degree in Physical Therapy from an accredited institution and approval by the American Physical Therapy Association. Must be currently state licensed as a physical therapist.

III. Duties:
   A. Administrates and implements patient care.
      1. Performs an initial evaluation of patients when ordered.
      2. Prepares and implements a treatment plan in agreement with patients' evaluation data, diagnosis, and prognosis, and doctors' orders.
      3. Therapeutically performs physical and chemical agents, exercise and other procedures to minimize pain and maintain independence.
      4. Assesses the rehabilitative status and makes recommendations on a regular, weekly basis.
      5. Performs treatment plans as ordered by the physicians.

   B. Maintains patient documentation according to departmental policy and procedures.
      1. Makes documentation in patient records on the summary of evaluations, reasons for referral, goals and problems, etc.

2. Consults with physicians, nurses, and other allied health personnel on treatment plans.
3. Records progress notes on patient's goals.
4. Records home instructions, discharge summaries and follow-up care.

C. Communicates with patients, employees, supervisors, and physicians to provide appropriate information.
   1. Discusses procedures and goals with patients prior to treatment.
   2. Consults with physicians regarding patient treatment.
   3. Reports to the physician and nurses all unusual reactions of patients.
   4. Instructs patient and family members in follow-up care and provides written instructions as needed.
   5. Conducts department and quality assurance committee meetings monthly to discuss new developments and programs.
   6. Attends interdisciplinary patient care meetings.

D. Assumes responsibility for administrative functions in the physical therapy department.
   1. Maintains a current manual consisting of departmental policies and procedures.
   2. Reviews annual departmental policies and procedure manuals.
   3. Plans department expenses and budgets.
   4. Completes employee evaluations annually.
   5. Supervises the patient care programs.
   6. Complies with safety standards and quality control.
   7. Develops infection control standards.
   8. Provides staff orientation programs, in-service training, continuing education programs, and documents and distributes material.
   9. Attends departmental managerial meetings and hospital interdepartmental meetings.
   10. Provides in-service and educational programs to hospital staff and community, as needed or requested.
   11. Reviews productivity and performance of staff.

E. Maintains competency in the profession by various means including continuing education programs.

F. Complies with and enforces hospital rules and regulations.

7. Another highly effective strategy is *organizing an effective advertising campaign* by utilizing these methods:

A. Place openings in *help wanted advertisements* in newspapers and other sources of media. (Please refer to Chapter 2, pages 45-46; and Appendix-References/Resources; pages 167-169.)

B. Use *direct mail techniques* to reach physical and occupational therapists in their homes.

C. *Secure paid or donated radio-TV time.* Select as best as possible the stations most likely heard by therapists and keep your message simple and easy to understand. Announce your staff opportunities in any media appearances.

Advertised openings can produce a favorable response and needs to be written, announced, and placed in the most effective way to attract candidates. Use of an advertising agency can assist you in providing an effective image by saving you time and money. An advertising agency can provide you surveys and skills in preparing your campaign.

All advertising should be honest and bona-fide openings. The variety of advertisement forms discussed in Chapter 2 (pages 45-46) are all types you need to be careful of not placing. Also the employer needs to understand the legal requirements in hiring that adversely affects people based on race, religion, national origin, age, sex, marital status, or physical handicaps. (See Chapter 6—Employer's Legal Requirements.) Some terms and phrases not to use are: "age 25 to 35," "college student," "recent college graduate," or other expressions of similar discriminatory nature.

A few helpful tips to consider when placing advertisements are:

• The best day of the week for newspapers to receive a higher response is Sunday. The Sunday edition usually carries the most job openings.

• List the job in the correct heading such as "Director of Physical Therapy," or "Occupational Therapist," and not in headings such as "Healthcare Professional,"

"Manager of Healthcare," or any other non-specific title, which a physical or occupational therapist may not look at.

• Try to include in your advertisement, if your budget will allow it, either a toll-free number or the term "Call Collect." List the phone number along with a specific employer representative. It is important to properly instruct your staff, including your answering service, switchboard personnel, and secretaries the importance of receiving any "Call Collects" which may come in. The response rate will be higher for you when you pay for the calls, especially for out-of-town applicants.

8. It is generally suggested that *offering competitive salaries and benefits* will attract and retain good therapists from the outset. If it is fiscally possible, increase the salaries and benefits if you are not competitive and review the cost of living increases. This may save your organization time and money in high turnover and recruitment expenses. In reviewing factors in recruiting and retaining staff, see Figure 13: Outline of Factors to Review with Therapists; also see the Appendix-Salary Surveys. How does your facility compare to these figures?

9. Another suggestion for positive recruitment and retention of staff is *committing to educational programs,* including courses, seminars, conferences, and in-service. Therapists need new information and educational information to stay abreast in their careers. In-service programs should include staff from other disciplines and occasional visiting specialists. Hosting seminars may even attract therapists from other facilities to consider working for your facility by this exposure. Tuition reimbursement is appealing to young therapists with minimal degrees but is also attractive to the physical therapy profession, which recently has passed a motion to lengthen the educational requirements beyond the bachelor's degree. Many occupational therapists, as well, attend educational courses every year to obtain a master's degree or to expose themselves to career advancement and knowledge. Sponsoring at least one educational

course per year by alloting money and time for that purpose supports the employer's willingness in recognizing the value of education.

10. Another educational incentive employers are promoting is *awarding scholorships and/or stipends to students* in exchange for a specified work period. This enhances the recruitment of therapists and builds loyalty to the employer. For example, Hospital XYZ has sponsored full tuition to Bill Jones, a senior occupational therapist, for his senior year of college. In return Bill Jones has agreed to work as an occupational therapist for two years of full-time employment at Hospital XYZ, after his graduation.

11. Similarly, many managers achieve recruitment value by *making professional presentations* and by *publishing articles* in recognized journals. Through such efforts, physical therapy and occupational therapy department heads sell their professionalism and market the quality of their department and facility to potential applicants.

12. Because professional development is very important to therapists, managers can *allow senior staff members to teach at local universities.* Freeing your staff to teach a few hours a week on company time is an effective way to recruit potential staff. The students learn about your facility, and you can use your experience to teach them.

13. Some employers also *sponsor student clinical education programs* that provide practical experience and attract promising students—who provide a potential source for therapists at a later date. By providing a challenging and stimulating environment, employers often retain many of the students after graduation. Large university affiliated hospitals generally hire more than *half* of their therapy staff from student clinical programs, reported Pamela Hooper in *Clinical Management* (1985, No. 2). At the same time, these programs contribute to increased staff productivity.

14. Other employers of therapists cooperate with area colleges in *developing work-study programs* and offer financial stipends in return for work. Students can function in part-

time and temporary positions and provide added exposure to the facility. Hands-on experience to these students promotes students to be recruited in entering physical and occupational therapy schools.

15. Within the employer's organization, a highly effective strategy can produce results in hiring employees— *recruiting informally by word of mouth.* According to Kathleen Gerber and Mary Ann Dettman in *Physical Therapy Bulletin* (July 30, 1986), "word of mouth," was the favorite source of information physical therapists used in their employment search. The employer can also tap the network of professional groups, such as local, state, and national associations. Frequently, positions are posted at conferences or workshops or at colleges and universities.

16. *Offering interviewing and relocation expenses, plus sign-on bonuses* enhances the employers' odds of attracting and hiring therapists. The employers' chances of obtaining staff by assisting with the interviewing and relocation expenses is an attractive added incentive for out-of-town candidates. As long as there is an increasing competitive climate, conducting recruitment as "business-as-usual" with no attractive incentives, will not usually work too long. If the employer's recruitment budget will not allow for full interviewing costs, negotiate an offer of the expenses to satisfy the candidate. Many times employers will specify interviewing expenses are provided in full or partial reimbursement if the candidate is hired and retained for at least one year of employment. Also relocation assistance and sign-on bonuses are often specified as conditional upon one year of employment.

17. Out-of-town candidates are attracted to employers *providing housing for a specified time,* either at no cost or at minimal cost to the employee. Relocation may be a smoother transition for candidates when nearby housing is provided from one to six months or longer. If the housing is in close proximity to the facility this further assists the candidate in enabling him or her to walk to work, particularly for the new graduate, who may be lacking transportation.

112

18. Many employers *attend career fairs and sponsor open houses.* This not only serves as an effective marketing technique but it exposes the services to the public, and announces available job opportunities to prospective candidates. Career fairs often are held at conferences, colleges and universities, and health care expositions. Normally a booth is assigned to the employer for the purpose of literature display and employer representation. Open houses can be announced in advertisements in any of the advertising methods—"help wanted" advertisements, direct mail to therapists' homes, or on radio-TV time. Often open houses serve refreshments including beverages such as coffee, tea, or punch along with cookies to provide a hospitable, relaxed atmosphere in promoting positive recruitment.

19. Some employers elect to use *professional recruiting agencies* in assisting with their recruiting. Recruiting firms can save time and offer a pool of available candidates, readily accessible for interviewing and hiring (see Chapter 2 — Employment Agencies-pages 47-49).

20. *International recruitment* has been providing a solution to staffing strategies. Seeking therapists outside the country and recruiting them to the United States increases the supply of therapists. These foreign educated, English-proficient, bachelor-degree-equivalent physical and occupational therapists require the facility to sponsor them. The guidelines set forth by the United States Department of Immigration and Naturalization Service as well as the foreign country's immigration department must be followed. Due to the complexity of the paperwork involved with immigration, it is suggested that the employer seek the assistance of an experienced employment agency or an experienced contract company.

Figure 13: **Outline of Employee Concerns**

This outline includes factors for the rehabilitation employer to be aware of in retaining and recruiting employees. Employers need to stay on the competitive edge and know what employees look for, either while they are employed with you or interviewing with you. If your facility is struggling to recruit employees with no luck, perhaps a review of these factors needs your attention. The more incentives you can offer an employee, the higher your odds in securing staff!

1. *Position*
   Title
   Job description
   Growth potential
   Budget-actual and projected
   Supervisors, peers,
      subordinates
   Reason position is open

2. *Company*
   Size of company, anticipated
      growth
   Specialties in industry
   Reputation
   Travel, if required
   Service population and area
      services
   Philosophy of care
   Financial report

3. *Equipment*
   Modern
   Outdated
   Maintenance

4. *Facility Appearance*
   Ample space
   Professional
   Clean
   Neat

5. *Patients*
   Types (general, acute, etc.)
   Number
   Occupancy
   Age

6. Size of staff
   Rehabilitation department
   Physicians

   Allied health
   Other

7. *Employees*
   Personality of office
   Conservative
   Liberal
   Friendly
   Enthusiastic
   Relaxed
   Number of minorities

8. *Location*
   Ease of travel
   Public transportation
   Distance from home
   Safety

9. *New location* (if relocating)
   Housing
   Schools, college, universities
   Climate
   Cultural activities
   Recreational activities
   Job opportunities for spouse
   Taxes—local, state, federal
   Cost of living
   Places of worship—churches,
      synagogues, etc.

10. *Relocation assistance*
    Moving costs
    Trips to locate new home
    Housing provided for
       specified time

11. *Interviewing costs*
    Interview assistance
    Second interview paid for
    Spouse trip paid

12. *Salary*
    Starting salary
    Salary potential
    Incentive, cost-of-living
      increases
    Sign-on bonus
13. *Fringe benefits*
    Health insurance—individual
      family, major medical,
      disability, prescriptions
    Dental
    Optical
    Holidays, personal days off
    Vacation
    Pensions/profit sharing
    Company car
    Social activities
    Professional dues

Meeting expenses
Uniforms provided and
  cleaned
Low interest loans
Discounted meals
Parking fees
Day care program
14. *Education programs*
    Seminars, conferences,
      courses
    In-service
    Student clinical
    Work-study
15. *Work schedule*
    Part-time
    Job sharing
    Flexible scheduling

Contracting Companies: A Staffing Alternative

Many facilities are participating in contractual agreements as an alternative to their personnel shortages in the rehabilitation unit, according to Deborah L. Stengel in *Clinical Management* (1986, No. 6, and 1987, No. 7). Physical and occupational therapy departments are contracting with outside management companies not only due to the shortage of therapists but also because they have found this alternative may help them to save on costs and run a more efficient department.

Contract companies first began in health care in non-clinical areas, such as laundry, housekeeping, food service, and materials management. (See Figure 14: Hospital Contract Management Services.) These contract services arose because of shortages of equipment or space, inefficient departments, turnover, or excessive costs. Contracted services may help the facility in controlling costs, increasing profits and providing services.

A variety of specialty programs are provided by contract companies. These include staff recruitment in areas such as orthopedics, pediatrics, sports medicine, back injury, geriatrics, industrial medicine, cardiology, and others. The companies can be national, local, or regional.

While therapists provide "hands on" service and assist in developing the patient plan, it is necessary for the health care facilities to control and monitor the service agreement with the contract company in order to maintain quality care for the patients. The contractual employees may be confused when first entering the new facility and in attempting to participate in the patient care plan. Therefore, good communications between the facility and the contracting agency employees will assist in solving problems and in maintaining a smooth transition. Because the contracting therapist is not an employee of the facility, authority issues often result. A job description clarifying the lines of authority should be determined in initial contract negotiations.

Figure 14: **Hospital Contract-Management Services**

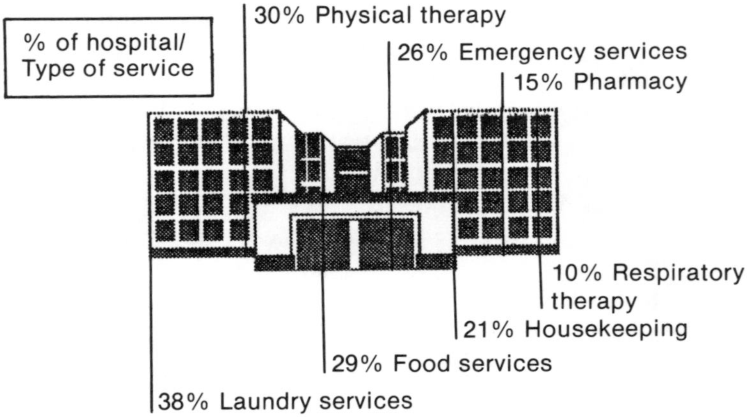

% of hospital/
Type of service

30% Physical therapy
26% Emergency services
15% Pharmacy
10% Respiratory therapy
21% Housekeeping
29% Food services
38% Laundry services

Source: American Hospital Publishing, Inc. survey of 400 hospitals in conjunction with HPI Health Care Services, Inc., 1987

Reprinted from *AHA News,* Vol. 24, No. 19, by permission, May 9, 1988, Copyright 1988, American Hospital Publishing.

Another helpful tactic is to provide an orientation period for contracting therapists in order for them to become familiar with the facility and to develop a carry-over system. Also, at the initial contract meeting, discussion of performance appraisals by management should be determined in consideration of further contract negotiations. Both the facility and the contracting company need to communicate information and decide upon mutual working agreements.

Employing Physical Therapy Assistants and Occupational Therapy Assistants

As the crisis continues with the shortage of occupational and physical therapists, employers have been recognizing and utilizing the services physical and occupational therapists provide. Both types of assistants function under the guidance of physical and occupational therapists to carry out treatment programs for many different kinds of patients. (Please refer to Figure 11: Traditional Organization Layout.)

The American Occupational Therapy Association and the American Physical Therapy Association both report a good outlook for assistants. The programs for these assistants are offered by community and junior colleges, and vocational/technical schools throughout the United States. Most programs lead to an associate degree and include practical experience in health care facilities. Graduates are eligible to take examinations to become certified. The physical therapy assistants take state examinations to become certified, while the occupational therapy assistants have a national examination to become certified.

Both the occupational and physical therapy assistants can help meet the demand in clinics, hospitals, rehabilitation centers, schools and nursing centers. Employers' recognition of these valuable contributors to health care can reduce the pressure of the rehabilitation department. Many times these assistants continue their careers further to become therapists while employed.

Can an understaffed rehabilitation facility continue to provide quality care employing only therapists when months go by with no physical or occupational therapists on the horizon to interview? Most employers will agree the answer to this is "No." Hiring assistants to help the therapists can be a practical solution and whenever applicable, they can provide a vital link to the rehabilitation team.

To learn more about the occupational therapy assistant program you may contact the occupational therapy schools nearby, the occupational therapy department in a local health care facility, or write or call:

The American Occupational Therapy Association, Inc.
1383 Pickard Drive
P.O. Box 1725
Rockville, MD 20850-4375

(301) 948-9626

Further information about the physical therapy assistant program can be obtained from the physical therapy schools nearby, the physical therapy department in a local health care facility, or write or call:

The American Physical Therapy Association, Inc.
1111 North Fairfax Street
Alexandria, VA 22314

(703) 684-2782

CHAPTER 6:

The Employer's Administrative Functions

- The Selection Process: Six Stages
    1. Screening
    2. Ranking
    3. Interviewing and Detailed Interview Topics
    4. Checking References
    5. Making the Final Hiring Decision
    6. Making the Job Offer
- Employer's Legal Requirements
    Pre-Employment Inquiry
- Employee Orientation
- Performance Reviews
    Sample Performance Review
- Termination of Employment
    1. Giving the Employee Warning
    2. Rules of Etiquette When Terminating

CHAPTER 6
The Employer's Administrative Functions

Selection Process

Much too often, employers seek the "perfect person" they hold out for the "perfect" applicant who never comes. Employers who are experienced in the selection process look for the "best" person available for the position. They take time to identify the position requirements, duties, and objectives, and find someone who can accomplish what is needed.

Managers rate the qualifications of various candidates as quickly as possible in order to choose the therapist most likely to be successful in the position. In order to be cost effective, the employer must get the new therapist "on board" without delay. The best candidate will be lost to another organization if the selection process goes on too long.

This usually means that candidates are measured against well developed criteria for a position, and are analyzed with regard to skills, possible length of stay, and other specific qualifications. For example, an orthopedic physical therapy coordinator should have experience in orthopedics and past management experience and an interest in management. Using good judgment and common sense, managers qualify each position function and recruit candidates with those skills.

For the applicant, the selection process starts with the first interview, and ends with the employer's decision. However, for the employer, the process is a succession of hurdles that begin with a present or future vacancy. The employer reviews the job description, consults with Equal Employment Opportunity department, and formulates a plan to recruit and interview candidates for the position.

The selection process usually has six stages:

1. Screening
2. Ranking
3. Interviewing
4. Checking References
5. Making the Final Selection
6. Making a Job Offer

As we will proceed to review the stages of the selection process from the screening to making a job offer, please refer to page 87, Figure 10: Positives and Negatives of Job Interviews. You can evaluate your candidates by using the positives and negatives listed.

Screening

Experienced managers screen each applicant quickly and immediately inform those who lack the necessary qualifications that they are not being considered for the position. This does not mean that applicants who fail to qualify for a present position may not be effective in another work situation, so managers often keep their applications on file.

Screening methods—through a personnel department or a recruiting agency should be closely monitored by managers who want to be successful in attracting top candidates. Organizations cannot afford to have qualified applicants eliminated from consideration. Many employers know that it is better to interview a candidate who might appear to be "borderline" rather than risk losing a qualified person based on an arbitrary decision.

Often managers use the phone to narrow down a large field of applicants. In this case, phone conversations become mini-interviews for the purpose of screening. This is especially important if candidates are located miles away and will have to travel far to be interviewed in person. In this way, managers often determine if they want to bring in out-of-town candidates.

Ranking

Managers then face the task of ranking applicants on how well each candidate met the predetermined criteria. In addition, interviewers or managers have to know and follow employment regulations. (See Employer's Legal Requirements, page 131-132.)

Employers who attract only a few candidates usually see all of them. However, if many applicants apply for the same position, managers have to select the most desirable for interviews.

This selection can be done by using the following ranking scale:

A. Unacceptable—They do not possess the minimum degree of skills needed for the position.

B. Marginal—They appear to possess the required degree of skills for the position.

C. Acceptable—They possess more than the marginal degree of skills.

D. Superior—Candidate displays a high degree of skills.

Interviewing

In the selection process, employers know that the interview is the critical stage—because that is when candidates form opinions of the manager and of the organization. It is also the time when employers and candidates get to know each other.

In order to present a well organized image, experienced managers tend to follow by the following guidelines:

1) Candidates should be informed in advance about the interview process, how long it will take, and who will be involved.

2) Enough time should be allowed for the candidate to tour the facility and obtain an overview of the rehabilitation department and the entire hospital.

3) The personnel or human resources department should spend time with the candidate, reviewing the application, explaining benefits, and exchanging information.

4) Provide enough time between interviews so that the candidate does not feel rushed. A half hour to an hour is usually adequate time for the first interview.

5) Put candidates at ease so they are willing to reveal their thoughts, goals, qualifications, and interests.

Figure 15: **Characteristics of a Good Interviewer**

1. Has a logical sequence in interviewing candidates
2. Puts applicants at ease
   a. Provides comfortable surroundings
   b. Engages in small talk (the weather, an interesting point on your resume, sports, etc.)
3. Outlines what will be covered in the interview
4. Makes an objective decision despite subjective reactions to the candidate's appearance, personality, race, religion, or background
5. Is sensitive to the applicant's fears and anxieties
6. Describes the job, answers questions, uses open-ended questions, gives a tour of the facility, introduces candidate to staff (whenever appropriate), keeps track of time, records results on standard form
7. Makes the hiring decision without unnecessary delay

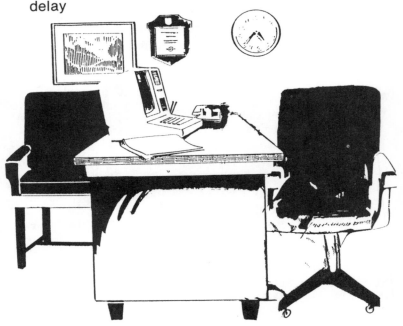

6) Give candidates a chance to express themselves, and keep the conversation open-ended. Do not ask questions that call for "yes" or "no" answers.

7) Give enough information about the facility and describe the staff and specialty areas, such as the pediatric ward, rehabilitation floor, or sports clinic. For example, "We have Scott Smith, PT, ATC., here for our sports medicine clinic and there are two therapists with him."

8) Give candidates time to answer and ask questions.

9) Use a standard form for recording interview results. Do not take detailed notes.

Detailed Interviewing Topics

Employers can discuss in detail questions that relate specifically to the candidate's prior education and work experience. Also the interviewer may discuss the applicant's attitudes and interests in physical or occupational therapy.

Recommended topics for discussion include:

A. Employment History
B. Job-Related Skills and Knowledge
C. Aptitude and General Intelligence
D. Attitudes and Personality
E. Educational and Training, Licenses

A. *Employment History* Candidates should be asked about their level of responsibility, earnings, and how their work relates to that of other therapists.

Managers often ask candidates the following questions:

"What was your position?"
"Why did you work there?"
"When did you work there?"
"How did you do the work?"
"Where did it happen?"
"Who was involved?"

Those who hire therapists look for gaps between positions and question time lapses. If an applicant has had a lot of experience, managers often concentrate on the earlier positions. These experiences mold people and tell something about who they are and who they want to be.

125

B. *Job Related Skills and Knowledge*   Here you are trying to determine the specifics of the candidate's prior employment; at what candidates did on the job; what types of activities they had; their level of responsiblity and the types of patient cases they treated on.

Typical questions to ask are:

"What types of patients did you treat at Jones Hospital?"

"How many therapists did you supervise?"

"As director of rehabilitation, what areas were you responsible for?"

C. *Aptitude and General Intelligence*   Based on how the candidate answers your questions in the interview, you can make a fair assumption concerning his/her general intelligence and aptitude. It is almost always a mistake to judge a candidate's aptitude or intelligence on the basis of appearance.

D. *Attitudes and Personality*   Usually during an interview, you can get an idea of what attitude the candidate has toward you, your facility and the job opening. By questioning the tasks he or she has done, you can develop an opinion about the candidate's personality. The manner in which he or she conducts himself can be characterized as appearing favorably, unfavorably, or indifferent. The more discussions you conduct, the more you will be able to determine his/her personal traits.

E. *Education, Training, and Licenses*   Managers know that a candidate's education, training, and licenses are important even though they may be a small part of the interview. Academic credits help to establish the applicant's attitude toward education. Confirmation of professional licenses is necessary for employment.

Many times, insight concerning a candidate's attitude toward continuing education and seminars can be determined during an interview discussion of education. Managers can ask about a candidate's interest in continuing education, seminars and conferences attended.

Checking References

The most effective recruiters check references over the phone, not through the mail. They know that they have to ask probing questions because most people tend to only say good things about past or present employees. Managers frequently talk to references from the candidate's present or previous place of work.

The key to successful reference checking is one's ability to convince the respondent that complete and candid information is in the best interest of the candidate as well as the employer. In checking references, recruiters most often describe the position that is available, and discuss the skills that will be needed.

Factual information that recruiters verify through reference checks are dates of employment, job titles, salary figures, reporting relationships, and reasons for the move. Work related references are more potent than academic ones because employers want tangible services.

Reference Check Questions

Typical questions when conducting reference checks include:

1) How long have you know the applicant?
2) How do you know the applicant?
3) Who hired the applicant?
4) What were his/her dates of employment?
5) What was the reason he/she left you?
6) What was his/her salary?
7) What was his/her job title and duties?
8) What was his/her absentee rate?
9) What was his/her attitude?
10) What was his/her appearance?
11) What were his/her patient skills?
12) Did he/she get along well with patients? Co-workers? Supervisors?
13) Was he/she dependable?
14) Did you have any problems with (the applicant)?
15) Is he/she eligible for rehire?

16) Did he/she need much supervision?

17) May I call you again for further information, if needed, or may someone else confirm this information with you?

Student Reference Checks

Regarding student applicants, employers frequently evaluate the student's transcript and clinical affiliations. Actually, grades provide a more accurate summary of performance than a faculty member's memory.

A common approach to student reference checks is provided on the following page: Reference Form—New Graduate.

Final Hiring Decision and Job Offer

After a manager has interviewed all of the candidates and identified his or her choice, that decision has to be made known as quickly as possible to the selected person. Waiting too long to extend an offer can risk your chance of securing the employee. It is not unusual for one to three months to pass before extending a job offer for a supervisory position. However, making an offer to a staff therapist can be done the same day as the interview (assuming the candidate meets your selection criteria).

Successful employers make their offers fair and competitive in terms of salary and benefits. The employer should be aware of the market value of comparable positions. This requires looking at salary surveys and job description along with advertisements in trade publications. Advertisements show compensation and positions nationally. (See Appendix-Salary Surveys.)

Employers look at the following factors in making an offer to top candidates:

- Total salary package—wages and benefits
- Salary surveys of physical/occupation therapists
- Financial need and revenue generating impact
- Employed past history of salaries and benefits
- Applicant's past history of salaries and benefits
- How long has this position been open?
- What is the policy on salary reviews and the cost of living expenses?

128

Reference Form—New Graduate

Scale of 1 to 10 (10 = highest)

1. Attendance _____
2. Dependability _____
3. Attitude _____
4. Quality of work _____
5. Appearance _____

Supervision of student (check one)

☐ Normal for a new graduate
☐ Needs more than average
☐ Does not need much

Did you have any particular problem that we should be aware of?

_____

_____

Name of reference _____

Title of Person _____

Name of facility _____

Address of facility _____

_____

Phone number of facility _____

Type of facility (check one)

☐ Hospital   ☐ Home care
☐ Free standing clinic ☐ Nursing home
☐ School   ☐ Other

Name of person who took this reference _____

Title of person _____

Date taken _____

Sample Cover Letter of Offer

St. Mary's Hospital
398 Main Street
New Town, Georgia 39482

June 4, 19XX

Mr. Mark Smith
7563 Jones St.
Atlanta, Georgia 48298

Dear Mark:

It was a pleasure to meet with you last week. In discussing your interview with Mr. Roberts, Director of Rehabilitation Services, we are quite impressed with your academic and clinical preparation for our position, as well as your personal attributes.

We would like to formally offer you a position as staff physical therapist at an annual salary of $XX,XXX, plus benefits listed on the yellow outline sheet, with relocation expenses of $X,000. Your benefits go into effect at your starting date of employment.

Should you accept our offer, we will be happy to help you with housing. We can make appointments for you to visit some apartments near the hospital, if you wish. We can also send you listings in the newspaper of housing opportunities available in the area.

As we discussed at the time of your interview, your employment is contingent upon successful completion of our physical examination, which we can schedule at your convenience. Your starting date of employment, which was late August or early September, is agreeable to us.

Again, it was a pleasure interviewing you on May 28, 19XX. We are hopeful that you will accept our offer. Please get in touch with me or Mr. Roberts at (404) 239-8943 on any questions or concerns you may have.

We look forward to your reply soon.

Sincerely,

Janis Walker
Employment Manager
cc: Jack Roberts, Director of Rehabilitation

130

- How much in a hurry is the facility to fill this position?
- How difficult has it been to interview other candidates?
- What salary did the previous person have?
- Are the times good for an increased salary for this position?

Employers usually contact candidates by phone to make an offer and then follow it up with a confirmation letter. The letter of confirmation should include:

- Title of the position and responsibility
- Starting salary
- Supervisor's name and phone number
- Benefits and when they are effective
- Relocation assistance, as authorized and needed
- Statement indicating employment is contingent upon successful physical examination
- Approximate starting date

For best results, this letter should be sent immediately to the candidate's residence. The previous page is an example of a letter of offer to a candidate. (Please also see Chapter 5, Figure 13: Outline of Factors to Review with Therapists, page 114.)

Employer's Legal Requirements

With the growing number of federal and state laws concerning discrimination in employment, legal issues in hiring are becoming an issue in the health care field. Personnel managers, as well as some physical and occupational therapy managers, need to be aware of these laws and the need for compliance.

Everyone involved in hiring should become familiar with the employment laws. Managers should know they can not set hiring standards that adversely affect people because of race, religion, national origin, age, sex, marital status, or physical handicap. If discrimination can be shown, institutions often are held responsible and financially accountable.

It makes no difference to government officials whether discrimination was the result of ignorance or of a prejudicial design. For instance, if a rehabilitation supervisor interviews a newly married woman and asks if she plans on having children soon, it is an illegal hiring question and is discriminatory, whether or not the supervisor recognizes the fact.

Donald S. Skupsky, JD, CRM, in *Recordkeeping Requirements,* states the legal requirements for employment records such as job applications, resumes, and advertising should be maintained for at least one year, according to the Age Discrimination Employment Act.

Certain questions are prohibited from being asked in an interview, nor can they appear on an application form. Anyone involved in hiring, as well as therapists applying for a position, should be aware of illegal questions. (See Figure 16: Pre-Employment Inquiry Guide.)

Employee Orientation

Beginning a new job can be stressful, almost a culture shock for the new employee, as well as an emotional experience. The first impression of a new position is usually quite lasting. The excitement and enthusiasm of the new employee should be well received by the employer, and be transmitted into loyalty from a satisfied physical or occupational therapist.

The employee should be greeted warmly, treated courteously, and handled professionally and efficiently. The new employee should learn the basic essentials of the facility, such as where to hang his or her coat, where the restrooms are located, where to eat lunch and other necessary pieces of information. However, if the new employee is handled indifferently, or receives a careless reception, he or she will view the new job with skepticism.

The objectives of the orientation period are to provide a pleasant working environment for the new employee and make him or her feel at ease. Hopefully the new employee will form a positive impression as the orientation continues which will help them blend into the workplace.

Another objective is to establish the feeling that the new employee really belongs and is an important member of the work group. When shown a sincere interest, he or she will adopt a team approach attitude and fit in with the co-workers.

The employee orientation also motivates and prepares the new employee for the future activities of the facility and of the department itself. Any changes, additions, etc., that are being worked on should be indicated to the new employee during this orientation period. For example, "Currently our department transports the rehab patients; however, within the next few weeks nursing staff will be handling this instead of us."

The four phases of employee orientation are:

1. The new employee meets someone from the department and is given information about the job, the facility, and the basic functions of the department, including patient services provided.

2. The new employee reports to his or her supervisor and the location he or she is to work. Here the new employee meets his or her fellow co-workers, learns where to hang his coat, where to eat, and all other personal details. Fellow co-workers conduct an informal orientation.

3. The personnel or human resources department conducts an orientation in a classroom setting. This may last for a period of weeks or months. This is where the company rules, policies, benefits, recreational and social activities are explained. There may be films, lectures, a company tour, or group meetings with other new employees.

4. The final phase is where the new employee is given final details of the more complex aspects of the job in his or her working area. This may be over a six month period. Here the new employee can discuss any concerns, problems, or questions about anything that has arisen during the first six months of work.

There is wide variation on the phases of the orientation and how information is presented to the employees. This depends on the size of the facility and how structured the environment may be. Finally, after the first six months, the new employee has completed the probationary period and should have a good understanding of the job routine.

Figure 16: **Pre-Employment Inquiries**

The Pre-Employment Inquiry Guide is based on the provisions of Public Acts 220 and 453 of 1976. The Michigan Department of Civil Rights developed this guide to assist employers and employment agencies in complying with both Acts in regards to pre-employment inquiries and certain data relating to job applicants. Other state statutes and regulations generally parallel this guide with a few variations. You should review the legal requirements for those states in which your institution does business.

SUBJECT	LAWFUL PRE-EMPLOYMENT INQUIRIES	UNLAWFUL PRE-EMPLOYMENT INQUIRIES
Name:	Applicant's full name.	Original name of an applicant whose name has been changed by court order or otherwise
	Have you ever worked for this company under a different name?	Applicant's maiden name.
	Is any additional information relative to a different name necessary to check work record? If yes, explain.	
Address or Duration of Residence:	How long a resident of this state or city?	
Birthplace:		Birthplace of applicant.
		Birthplace of applicant's parents, spouse or other close relatives.
		Requirement that applicant submit birth certificate, naturalization or baptismal record.
Age:	*Are you 18 years old or older?	How old are you? What is your date of birth?

*This question may be asked only for the purpose of determining whether applicants are of legal age for employment.

SUBJECT	LAWFUL PRE-EMPLOYMENT INQUIRIES	UNLAWFUL PRE-EMPLOYMENT INQUIRIES
Religion or Creed:		Inquiry into an applicant's religious denomination, religious affiliations, church, parish, pastor, or religious holidays observed.
		An applicant may not be told "This is a Catholic (Protestant or Jewish) organization."
Race or Color:		Complexion or color of skin.
Photograph:		Requirement that an applicant for employment affix a photograph to an employment application form.
		Request an applicant, at his or her option, to submit a photograph.
		Requirement for photograph after interview but before hiring.
Height:		Inquiry regarding applicant's height.
Weight:		Inquiry regarding applicant's weight.
Marital Status:		Requirement that an applicant provide any information regarding marital status or children. Are you single or married? Do you have any children? Is your spouse employed? What is your spouse's name?
Sex:		Mr., Miss or Mrs. or an inquiry regarding sex. Inquiry as to the ability to reproduce or advocacy of any form of birth control.

SUBJECT	LAWFUL PRE-EMPLOYMENT INQUIRIES	UNLAWFUL PRE-EMPLOYMENT INQUIRIES
Health:	Do you have any impairments, physical, mental, or medical which would interfere with your ability to do the job for which you have applied?	Inquiries regarding an individual's physical or mental condition which are not directly related to the requirements of a specific job and which are used as a factor in making employment decisions in a way which is contrary to the provisions or purposes of the Michigan Handicappers' Civil Rights Act.
	Inquiry into contagious or communicable diseases which may endanger others. If there are any positions for which you should not be considered or job duties you cannot perform because of a physical or mental handicap, please explain.	Requirement that women be given pelvic examinations.
Citizenship:	Are you a citizen of the United States?	Of what country are you a citizen?
	If not a citizen of the United States, does applicant intend to become a citizen of the United States?	Whether an applicant is naturalized or a native-born citizen; the date when the applicant acquired citizenship.
	If you are not a United States citizen, have you the legal right to remain permanently in the United States? Do you intend to remain permanently in the United States?	Requirement that an applicant produce naturalization papers or first papers.
		Whether applicant's parents or spouse are naturalized or native-born citizens of the United States; the date when such parent or spouse acquired citizenship.
National Origin:	Inquiry into languages applicant speaks and writes fluently.	Inquiry into applicant's (a) lineage; (b) ancestry; (c) national origin; (d) descent; (e) parentage, or nationality.
		Nationality of applicant's parents or spouse.
		What is your mother tongue?
		Inquiry into how applicant acquired ability to read, write or speak a foreign language.

136

SUBJECT	LAWFUL PRE-EMPLOYMENT INQUIRIES	UNLAWFUL PRE-EMPLOYMENT INQUIRIES
Education:	Inquiry into the academic, vocational or professional education of an applicant and the public and private schools attended.	
Experience:	Inquiry into work experience. Inquiry into countries applicant has visited.	
Arrests:	Have you ever been convicted of a crime? If so, when, where and nature of offense? Are there any felony charges pending against you?	Inquiry regarding arrests.
Relatives:	Names of applicant's relatives, other than a spouse, already employed by this company.	Address of any relative of applicant, other than address (within the United States) of applicant's father and mother, husband or wife and minor dependent children.
Notice in Case of Emergency:	Name and address of person to be notified in case of emergency.	Name and address of nearest relative to be notified in case of accident or emergency.
Military Experience:	Inquiry into an applicant's military experience in the Armed Forces of the United States or in a State Militia. Inquiry into applicant's service in particular branch of United States Army, Navy, etc.	Inquiry into an applicant's general military experience.
Organizations:	Inquiry into the organizations of which an applicant is a member excluding organizations, the name or character of which indicates the race, color, religion, national origin or ancestry of its members.	List all clubs, societies and lodges to which you belong.
References:	Who suggested that you apply for a position here?	

Performance Reviews

The performance review helps provide solutions to management problems such as dealing with salary increases, promotions from within, and training. They serve in helping to format suggestions for improving future performance. Most reviews examine performance on traits such as:

1. Organization
2. Planning
3. Rapport with patients and employees
4. Initiative and cooperation
5. Written communication
6. Leadership

A performance review system tells employees what is expected of them, how well they are doing, and what the employer can do to enhance their performance. It gives an indication of what an employee can do to modify his or her work behavior in order to become a more effective performer.

A performance review system also tells a manager how his or her staff is performing in such areas as:

1. Potential for leadership
2. Overall evaluation
3. Necessary improvement
4. Outstanding ability
5. Relationship with subordinates, peers, and supervisors
6. Areas needing improvement

When conducting a performance review session, the meeting should be set in a quiet office, not in the middle of the department or staff office. Try to make the conversation a dialogue, and try to keep it pleasant. It is a good time to discuss goals for the coming year, and to discuss ways to obtain these goals. The topics of continuing education, conferences and seminars are appropriate to discuss at this time as well. See the following page for a Sample Performance Review.

Sample Performance Review

Employee _____ Department _____

Supervisor _____ Date _____

Type of Review: ☐ 60 days
☐ semiannual
☐ yearly

	Above Average	Fair	Poor
Quality of work			
Quantity of work			
Job Knowledge			
Judgment			
Cooperation			
Attitude			
Appearance			
Communication with Patients			
Communication with Employees			
Attendance			
Adaptability			
Dependability			
Leadership			

_____   _____
Employee Signature   Supervisor's Signature

_____
Date

Termination of Employment

Terminating an employee's services graciously requires the employer's best managerial skills. Most managers abhor the thought of letting anyone go. Yet, it may be the biggest favor a boss can do for a person who is not working out. Despite all the care taken in the selection process, mistakes can be made. A therapist may possess all the necessary technical skills and still not be effective in a particular work situation. The person may not fit into the philosophy of the organization.

Give the Employee Warning

The terminated employee may expect to be dismissed, and it may not come as a surprise. Most facilities have a terminating policy, in writing, which is part of the orientation kit given to each employee. The policy should be detailed enough to cover any situation which could be cause for dismissal.

It is important to communicate dissatisfaction with an employee's performance before terminating him or her. One way to do this is to establish a time limit for improvement. Inform the employee what is expected in the way of improvement and when it is expected.

Rules of Etiquette With Termination

All conversations should be kept confidential between the manager and the employee. This issue should not be discussed when other employees are in the office. When dismissing someone, the manager should keep it quiet until the person being dismissed has been told.

Likewise, it is important to show respect for an employee who is being terminated. Tell the person what he or she has done wrong, but do not make a long speech about it. In order to justify the decision, the manager should have on hand necessary records, forms, or evaluations.

Other factors to be considered include the following:

• The method of transferring medical and life insurance policies should be explained to the employee.

• A statement of any profit and pension plan benefits should be given to the employee.

• Legal issues may occur when there is an employment contract or an accused unjust dismissal. Giving employees ample warnings and recording the warnings often protects management against discrimination charges. Also, employers should draw attention to job performance, not the employee's personality. Leave the mud-slinging to politicians.

• If giving a recommendation, indicate the person's good points, even though the person was discharged. Negative comments must be said tactfully.

• Termination should be done in person and not in writing or over the phone.

CHAPTER 7
Conclusion

- Post-Search Networking and Self-Examination
- Tips on Succeeding in Your New Job Assignment
- How to Get the Salary You Deserve
- What to Do if Your New Job Isn't Working Out

CHAPTER 7
Conclusion

As rehabilitation professional shortages have become widespread, it is time for employers to be openminded towards changes in methods of hiring staff. This book does not guarantee success but it has increased your odds for success and broadened your knowledge. It is up to you to use this knowledge to best suit your needs.

For the physical and occupational therapists, this book has presented a practical guide on how to be hired—from the pre-search process to the post-search steps. At the end of this chapter you will find for your review a job search checklist, salary surveys, network logs, list of references/resources, and the bibliography. I recommend to both the employer and employee that you seek out further information listed in the appendix.

There is a job out there that you will enjoy, if you are the employee. For the employer, there is a candidate to fill your job opening. The job search process for both the employee and the employer may take longer than you first anticipated, but the fact that you have read this book displays your interest in improving your organization or your situation by seeking advice and examining many available options.

Your attitude is a key factor and will help your odds despite the increasing job market demands. A person displays an attitude of a two-way street if he or she asks, "How can I help myself or facility become better?" You generally receive what you give back in return. A poor attitude is apparent to others and can affect your success. If you take the steps you should, spend the time it will need and not let yourself get discouraged, you will succeed. Remember, there is no "perfect" job and there is no "perfect" applicant. If you believe you can improve your current situation, it will happen.

Now, let us assume that you are the employee and your job hunt is over and you have just started to work in your new position. There are two areas that need attention: Post-search networking and self-examination.

Post-Search Networking

You have a lot of time, energy, and money in developing your job search network. It is a good idea to maintain your contacts for future career advancement or in the event you may have a problem with your new job. No position is ever guaranteed for life, whether it is a new job or one of long standing.

Some suggestions for maintaining your network are:

1. Send your thank-you notes to everyone on your network list. It is important to write thank-you notes to the people who sincerely tried to help you or directed some interest and kindness your way. Thankful recognition should be shown for the help you received—help which you may need again sometime. Do not forget to write to friends, personnel managers, employment counselors and anyone else who has helped you. Taking a few minutes to thank them is simple courtesy and it just might pay off in the future.

2. Inform prospective employers about your new job after you have started it, not before. Until you start your new job, you may have to say you are in negotiations.

3. Besides thanking potential employers and network individuals, state that you would like to maintain contact. Then keep in touch with them periodically to find out what is new in their organization.

4. If you were in contact with recruiters or agencies, contact them again and inform them of your new position. You may then become a part of their "employed data base," and they may use *you* as a networking source. In this way, you will stay informed about new openings and the movement of your colleagues.

5. The individuals who provided references for you also need to be acknowledged with a thank-you note. Thank

them for their support and inform them of your new position.

6. Organize your network list and make sure it is on paper. Keep the name of the contact person, address, phone number, and any other notes in a file for future use.

7. Congratulate those in the spotlight—newspapers, radio, TV, etc. Be sure to congratulate individuals on your network list who receive favorable recognition in the news. You may be reading the *Occupational Therapy Forum,* a newspaper, or any other publication and spot news about those in your network. You may also see them as guest speakers or when they are conducting a seminar. They will be happy to hear from you, and you will maintain your contact. (See Appendix for Network Logs.)

In addition, you will want to review new knowledge about yourself and how you fit into the job market. This is not an idle exercise, but a dynamic and necessary part of your personal career advancement.

Self-Examination

Careful consideration of the following questions can assist you in evaluating your present status and help you identify future areas for personal development:

1. How can you improve yourself to become a better employee?

2. Why did you leave your last job? What went wrong?

3. Do you follow changes in the rehabilitation industry?

4. What techniques do you use to communicate effectively with patients, co-workers, and supervisors? If improvement is needed, what course of action should you take?

5. What new skills can you learn through your new job, education, seminars, reading and outside research?

Tips on Succeeding at Work

Of course you want to be successful in your new position. You want to prove that you can do the work to yourself, your family, your friends, and your employer. Here are a number of tips on succeeding in your new position:

1. *Conserve your energy at the beginning*   The first few weeks in a new position are stressful and will take more energy than you expect. Try not to commit yourself to a heavy social schedule, long weekend trips, or keeping late hours. You need to be alert and healthy and you need to get plenty of sleep.

2. *Ask questions*   Fear of appearing stupid is the reason most people do not ask questions. However, it is better to ask questions than to suffer serious results of mistakes. Do not interrupt a person who is very busy, especially if he or she is talking to someone. Wait for a convenient time to ask questions. If necessary ask for a replay so that you are sure that you clearly understand, and take notes—it can help. As Josh Billings once said: "The trouble with people is not that they don't know but they know so much that ain't so."

3. *Make friends, but not close friends too soon*   Other employees may be friendly the first few days when you begin your new job, but beware. Perhaps these "friendly" people are not respected by the others, and are trying to gain allies. This may result in putting you in a difficult situation. Building working relationships with all the people during the first few weeks is wise; don't spend all your time with only one or two employees.

4. *Be organized*   You will be presented with a lot of rules, procedures and important information at first. Keep a notebook and record these hard to remember facts. At night, review the facts and procedures. Employee handbooks and materials for new employees contain important information and should be reviewed also.

5. *Be positive*   A positive attitude toward your job, your employer and life in general will help you create a good impression. Nonverbal positive signals include shaking hands, opening doors for people, gesturing positively with the hand, and smiling. When you send out signals in good humor, others will not feel awkward about approaching you, and you will begin to build positive personal relationships.

6. *Be on time*   It is your responsibility to get to work on time, or even early. If you are depending on someone else for transportation, be sure he or she is responsible or make other

arrangements. If you drive, keep your car in good mechanical order; check your tires frequently and have sufficient gas. If you need to work late, do it cheerfully and without complaining.

How to Get the Salary You Deserve

What is a realistic way to get an increase? You need to start by asking yourself two questions:

1. How much am I worth?
2. How can I make myself worth more?

Your salary is determined by how well you perform, and what your performance level is worth to your organization. The key to getting what you deserve is to assure that your supervisor realizes what you do, how you do it, and what it is worth. This information is then considered as part of your salary review.

To begin with, determine if there is a formal policy concerning performance appraisals and salary reviews in your organization. A structured program for salary reviews often includes a specific time for review, as well as salary ranges and grade levels. You need to understand how this works, and know how often you are going to have a salary review. If there is no formal structure for salary reviews, try to establish one with your supervisor. See Figure 17 on specific steps you can take to get a salary review system working.

Remember, the salary review and performance appraisal are not the same thing. The performance appraisal is the best method of getting the money you want, not the salary review. If you work with your supervisor, you can develop continual appraisals of your performance.

If there is no formal structure for salary review or performance appraisal, chances are you will not have a valid job description, either. You then need to work one out. The job description's function is to:

1. Outline the duties of the job
2. Serve as a basis for job evaluation
3. Assure that all work is assigned and accountable

Figure 17: **Do's and Don'ts for Salary Reviews**

Salary Reviews—Some Useful Things to Do

1. Find out what the organization policy is concerning performance appraisals and salary reviews.
2. If there is no formal policy, try to establish one with your boss.
3. Try to separate your performance appraisal from your salary review procedure. Try to make the performance review a continual process.
4. Ask for written ground rules, when possible, on both performance appraisal times and standards, as well as salary review intervals.
5. Try to have your salary review at a good time for your organization (when profits are up, when they have just finished the peak season, after a successful new product introduction, etc.).

Salary Reviews—Some Precautions

1. Don't make your boss an adversary; use the performance review as a tool to ask for his or her help.
2. Don't make demands or threats.
3. Don't believe other employee's salary statements, or use them to support your case.
4. Don't take salary surveys and trade advertisements as gospel—each employee is a statistic of one!

Expectations *vs.* Performance

Aware of what was expected?	NO	How can criteria be made clear?
YES		
Aware of nonperformance?	NO	How can you become aware?
YES		
Encountered uncontrollable factors?	YES	How to avoid, eliminate, or accommodate?
NO		
Lack of ability?	YES	How to train?
NO		
Lack motivation?	YES	How to motivate?
NO		

Peringian, *Clinical Management,* 1984

4. Establish that you and your supervisor agree on what work is needed to be done

A good job description and performance appraisal helps you and your supervisor agree on how your performance will be measured before the salary review. Performance appraisals enable you to achieve goals and increase your ability and potential. They can help you realize the seven components to job success:

1. What is expected of you
2. What you expect of yourself
3. What your limitations are
4. Where you can get help
5. How to work without direction
6. How to improve your performance against your goal
7. Why and to what degree your salary increases should follow achievement

If you do not have job descriptions and appraisals, establish them and then your salary increases or your compensation should take care of itself.

There are several things you should *not* do:

1. Do not make your supervisor an adversary
2. Do not make demands or threats
3. Do not believe other employee's salary claims or use them to support your case
4. Do not take salary surveys and trade advertisements as the truth
5. Do not omit the factors considered in your salary program—cost of living, merit raises, longevity considerations, and incentive programs

In summation, try to have all the salary agreements, job descriptions, and performance appraisals in writing. Also, remember that if times are tough, it does not matter how good you are; a raise is *never* guaranteed. (See Appendix for Salary Surveys.)

What to Do if Your New Job Isn't Working Out

It makes no difference whether this is your first job out of college, or whether you have been in physical or occupational therapy for twenty years. The problem of taking a new job that does not work out happens to the best of us. The question to ask yourself is, "Why isn't my new job working out?" Examine the cause of your dissatisfaction. What expectations did you have that are not being met?

If your expectations are not being satisfied, find out reasons. Perhaps you are not getting the money and perks you anticipated. This type of problem can be resolved in a straightforward fashion by talking to the person who hired you.

Talk It Over

If you can be open with your supervisor regarding your concerns, that is the first person you should talk to. If not, you may be able to discuss the situation with a personnel representative, who should be experienced in handling monetary, psychological, and human relations problems. Other job related problems may not be that easy to explore.

The person you talk to might even provide information to help you make a decision. They may provide you with some "inside" information: you may discover that someone plans to retire, or that a new facility is opening, which may mean a promotion for you.

If you are at the early stages of your career, it is likely that whatever caused you to leave your previous position is behind your desire to change now. Reasons that make the physical or occupational therapy professional feel compelled to change employers are usually reflected in their new job expectations. Poor management is often a good reason given by therapists for leaving a position. Other reasons include undesirable relocation, no advancement opportunity, or lack of challenge.

If you are near retirement age, you may decide to stay and make the best out of the remaining time left with your employer. No matter what your situation, after expressing your concerns to a third party in the organization, you may still decide your job is not going to work out; the situation is intolerable. Whatever the reasons, you may decide to start looking at other options.

Do Not Quit

One option is to quit and look for another job. *Do Not Quit!* Start to look, but do not leave your job until you have another one lined up. The job market favors people who are employed, whether the economy is good or bad.

Begin your job search by updating your resume and contacting people from your network. This is also the time to contact past agencies and recruiters you worked with in the past, as well as organizations you interviewed with before.

Your Timetable

When studying market acceptance of professional job changes, there is a clearly defined timetable that must not be ignored. The basic rule of thumb is that you should ideally stay in your first job for at least three years, or at the very minimum, two years. The reason is that in physical or occupational therapy, you learn the job the first year, start handling it capably during the second year, and become really productive during the third year. If you have been a therapist for more than three years and have moved up to a directorship position, you should try to stay a total of six years in that position—three years for each of those two jobs.

If you make a change within the first six months but had three years in your previous job, the switch can be readily explained. After a few months on a job, it is possible to say, "The organization is not all that it was cracked up to be." However, such a reason is not as easily accepted if you wait six to twelve months. Just make sure you do not make another move that soon from your next job. Short periods of employment need to be separated by periods of longer job tenure.

The job change timetable (see Figure 18) indicates that a move after two to four years is better than a change after six to eight years. After three years in the same job, employees

Figure 18: **Job Change Timetable**

1. One job change after less than six months on the job can probably be easily explained.
2. A move after six to twelve months is not as easily explained and could cause problems.
3. A move after two to four years usually is better than after six to nine years on the same job.
4. Try not to make your first move in less than three years, your first two changes within four to six years.

Peringian, *Clinical Management,* 1986

usually begin to lose value to their employer and to other employers.

Here are some hints for changing jobs:

1. Always keep your resume current
2. Always maintain a good relationship with your last employer. You may want to go back or may need him or her for a reference.
3. Always emphasize your past accomplishments.
4. Never be unemployed. Stay employed during your job search.
5. Do not make too many moves too soon. Jumps of nine months here and six months there are a handicap.

After weighing and reviewing carefully the timing, and other factors affecting your decision, do not be afraid to change jobs if your new job just is not working out.

Appendix

- Job Search Checklist
- Salary Surveys
- Network Logs
  Personal Contacts
  Phone
  Mail
  Interview
  Follow-up
  Responses—Offers/Acceptances/Rejections
- Resources/References
- Bibliography

Job Search Checklist

Every physical and occupational therapist can enhance the effectiveness of his or her job search by following these guidelines:

I. *Actions to Take Before Your Interview:*

1. Write down your long and short-term goals and keep them updated—like an itinerary of a trip you are planning.

2. Evaluate your present position as objectively as possible, like a balance sheet with credits and debits.

3. Rate yourself on personal strengths and weaknesses.

4. Examine what you want to gain both professionally and personally from your next position.

5. Begin your job search "in your own backyard"—the place where people know you best.

6. Work the unpublished market through your own network of contacts and keep that network active.

7. Study the techniques for answering advertisements.

8. Consider the possibility of using professional recruiters.

9. Take the time to prepare effective cover letters and resumes.

10. Research the facilities and the employers.

II. *What to Do During the Interview:*

1. Check the time of your appointments and arrive five to ten minutes early.

2. Be enthusiastic.

3. Dress appropriately for your interviews.

4. Listen carefully.

5. Ask relevant questions.

6. Try to appear relaxed and leave nervous habits at home.

7. Summarize the main points at the end of the interviews.

8. State examples to support your statements.

9. Smile and act pleasant; be polite and courteous.

III. *Follow-Up Steps After Your Interviews:*

1. Send thank-you notes to the employers a few days after the interviews.

2. Send thank-you letters to your friends, business contacts and anyone on your network list who helped.

3. Organize your network list, including network logs.

4. Maintain a good positive attitude.

1988 Occupational Therapist Salary Survey

Region	Average Annual Salary	Average Experience (years)	Average Number Hours/Week	Average Number Patients/Day	Average Percent Last Raise	Average Job Change Frequency
Western	$35,043.23	10.71	43.52	5.96	5.66%	2.49
Midwest/Southern	$34,958.20	10.84	45.91	5.78	6.15%	2.27
Atlantic	$34,674.69	10.97	42.55	6.52	6.65%	2.29

Occupational Therapy Director Regional Breakdown
Source: *Occupational Therapy Forum*, Vol. IV, No. 14, April 10, 1989
Reprinted with permission

Region	Average Annual Salary	Average Experience (years)	Average Number Hours/Week	Average Number Patients/Day	Average Percent Last Raise	Average Job Change Frequency
Western	$29,035.16	7.97	41.33	10.40	5.43%	1.93
Atlantic	$28,899.73	7.14	40.69	10.69	5.77%	1.88
Midwest/Southern	$27,974.58	7.69	41.61	10.13	5.27%	1.85

Staff Occupational Therapist Regional Breakdown
Source: *Occupational Therapy Forum*, Vol. IV, No. 9, March 6, 1989
Reprinted with permission

1988 Physical Therapist Salary Survey

Region	Average Annual Salary	Average Experience (years)	Average Number Hours/Week	Average Number Patients/Day	Average Percent Last Raise	Average Job Change Frequency
Western	$41,367.69	12.86	45.64	12.75	8.21%	2.49
Midwest/ Southern	$41,270.30	12.74	46.33	12.2	5.83%	2.74
Midatlantic	$40,397.32	12.72	44.22	12.72	6.77%	2.74
Northeast	$37,766.80	13.93	42.79	9.28	6.33%	2.61

Physical Therapy Director Regional Breakdown
Source: *Physical Therapy Forum*, Vol. VIII, No. 8, February 27, 1989
Reprinted with permission

Midatlantic	$34,199.31	6.57	41.78	13.31	6.37%	1.74
Midwest/ Southern	$34,151.43	8.18	43.11	12.17	6.42%	1.79
Western	$33,745.60	8.39	42.54	12.17	5.76%	2.03
Northeast	$31,349.90	8.09	41.48	11.84	6.38%	1.74

Staff Physical Therapist Regional Breakdown
Source: *Physical Therapy Forum*, Vol. VIII, No. 14, April 10, 1989
Reprinted with permission

Personal Contacts

Date	Name	Company	Phone #

Phone Log

Date	Employer	Contact Person	Interest Y/N

Mail Log

Date	Employer	Contact Person	Source	Date for Follow-Up

Interview Log

Date	Employer	Contact Person	Status

Follow-Up Log

Date	Employer	Contact Person	Interest Y/N

Responses—Offers/Acceptances/Rejections

Date	Employer	Response	Comments

Resources/References

Newspapers
Local Newspapers
The New York Times
The Wall Street Journal

Directories
Allied Health Education Directory
American Medical Association
535 North Dearborn Street
Chicago, Illinois 60610

AHA Guide to the Healthcare Field
American Hospital Association
840 North Lake Shore Drive
Chicago, Illinois 60611

Organizations
American Academy of Health Administators
5530 Wisconsin Ave., NW
Washington, D.C. 20815

American College of Healthcare Executives
840 North Lake Shore Drive
Chicago, Illinois 60611

American Hospital Association
840 North Lake Shore Drive
Chicago, Illinois 60611

American Medical Association
535 North Dearborn Street
Chicago, Illinois 60610

American Occupational Therapy Association
1383 Piccard Drive
Rockville, Maryland 20850

American Osteopathic Hospital Association
212 East Ohio Street
Chicago, Illinois 60611

American Physical Therapy Association
1111 North Fairfax Street
Alexandria, Virginia 22314

Association of Mental Health Administrators
840 North Lake Shore Drive, Suite 1103 W.
Chicago, Illinois 60611

Commission on Accreditation of Rehabilitation Facilities
2500 North Pantano Road
Tucson, Arizona 85715

Department of Health and Human Services
National Institute of Mental Health
Division of Human Resources
5600 Fishers Lane
Rockville, Maryland 20857

National Association of Rehabilitation Facilities
P.O. Box 17675
Washington, D.C. 20015

National Easter Seal Society
70 East Lake Street
Chicago, Illinois 60611

National Rehabilitation Association
633 South Washington
Alexandria, Virginia 22314

Periodicals
The American Journal of Occupational Therapy
1383 Piccard Drive, P.O. Box 1725
Rockville, Maryland 20850-4375

Clinical Management in Physical Therapy
1111 North Fairfax Street
Alexandria, Virginia 22314

Hospitals
American Hospital Publishing, Inc.
211 East Chicago Ave.
Chicago, Illinois 60611

Journal of the American Physical Therapy Association
1111 North Fairfax Street
Alexandria, Virginia 22314

Occupational Therapy News
1383 Pickard Drive
Rockville, Maryland 20850-4375

Occupational Therapy Forum
251 West DeKalb Pk., Suite A-115
King of Prussia, Pennsylvania 19406

Occupational Therapy Week
3700 Wheeler Ave.
Alexandria, Virginia 22304

Physical Therapy Bulletin
3700 Wheeler Ave.
Alexandria, Virginia 22304

Physical Therapy/Occupational Therapy Job News
470 Boston Post Road
Weston, Massachusetts 02193

Physical Therapy Forum
251 West DeKalb Pk., Suite A-115
King of Prussia, Pennsylvania 19406

Today's Student Physical Therapist
American Physical Therapy Association
1111 North Fairfax Street
Alexandria, Virginia 22314

Bibliography

Bair, Jeanette; Gray, Madelaine. *The Occupational Therapy Manager.* The American Occupational Therapy Association, Rockville, MD. 1985, 223-226, 300-301.

Birsner, E. Patricia. *The 40 + Job Hunting Guide.* An Arco Book, Prentice Hall Press, New York, NY. 1987.

Bostwick, Burdette. *Resume Writing, A Comprehensive How-To-Do-It-Guide.* B.E. Bostwick Company Management Consultants, John Wiley and Sons, New York, NY. 1980.

Caple, John. *Careercycles.* Prentice-Hall, Inc., Englewood Cliffs, NJ. 1983.

Cebulski, Paulette; Sojkowksi, Marcia. "Clinical Education and Staff Profuctivity," *Clinical Management,* American Physical Therapy Association, VA. 1988, No. 4:26.

Ciccone, Charles; Wolfner, Michele. "Clinical Affiliations and Postgraduate Job Selection: A Survey," *Clinical Management.* American Physical Therapy Association, Alexandria, VA. 1988, No. 3:16-17.

Corwen, Leonard. *Your Resume: Key to a Better Job.* An Arco Book, Simon and Schuster, Inc., NY. 3rd Ed., 1988.

"Crisis Ahead," published by the Professional Advisory Council-National Easter Seal Society, August, 1988.

Dettman, Mary Ann; Gerber, Kathleen. "Facility Is Important Job Factor," *Physical Therapy Bulletin.* July 30, 1988:3.

Gerberg, Robert. *The Professional Job Changing System.* Performance Dynamics Publishing, Inc., NJ. 1981.

Half, Robert. *Robert Half on Hiring.* Crown Publishers, Inc., New York, NY. 1985

Hayes, Pamela. "A Change of Pace—Alternative Work Schedules Options," *Clinical Management.* American Physical Therapy Association, Alexandria, VA. 1989, No. 2:26-29.

Hooper, Pamela. "Recruitment—The Art of Being Prepared." *Clinical Management,* American Physical Therapy Association, Alexandria, VA. 1985, No. 2:36-37.

"Jobs in Allied Health Professions Are Plentiful," *AHA News.* American Hospital Association, Chicago, IL. July 18, 1988:2.

"AHA Tracks Shortages in Health Care Personnel," *AHA News.* American Hospital Association, Chicago, IL. January 2, 1989:1.

Occupational Outlook Handbook. U.S. Department of Labor, Washington, D.C., Bureau of Labor Statistics, April, 1988, Bulletin 2300; 1988-1989 Ed.

Peringian, Lynda. "My New Job Isn't Working Out," *Clinical Management.* American Physical Therapy Association, Alexandria, VA. 1986, No. 6:32-33.

Peringian, Lynda. "How to Get the Salary You Deserve," *Clinical Management.* American Physical Therapy Association, Alexandria, VA. 1984, No. 4:32-33.

Peringian, Lynda. "To Move or Not to Move," *Clinical Management.* American Physical Therapy Association, Alexandria, VA. 1985, No. 6:32-35.

Peringian, Lynda. "How to Explore the Job Market," *Clinical Management.* American Physical Therapy Association, Alexandria, VA. 1983, No. 4:46-47.

Peringian, Lynda. "How to Explore the Job Market," *Today's Student Physical Therapist.* American Physical Therapy Assocation, Alexandria, VA. Spring, 1989, 12-13.

Peringian, Lynda. "How to Get the Salary You Deserve," *Today's Student Physical Therapist.* American Physical Therapy Association, Alexandria, VA. Spring, 1989, 13-14.

Peringian, Lynda;Skeegan, Sam. "Attracting and Hiring the Right Person," *Clinical Management.* American Physical Therapy Association, Alexandria, VA. 1982, No. 3:11-12.

Peringian, Lynda; Skeegan, Sam. "Why Do Managers

Change Jobs?—Health Care Management," *Michigan Health Educator.* June, 1980, No. 3:11-12.

"Rehabilitation's Cost-Effectiveness Should Not Be Kept Secret Anymore," *AHA News,* American Hospital Association, Chicago, IL. July 11, 1988:4.

"Report Suggests Methods to Solve Physical Therapy Shortage," *Progress Report,* American Physical Therapy Association, Alexandria, VA. September 1988:4.

Skupsky, Donald S., JD, CRM, *Recordkeeping Requirements.* Information Requirements Clearinghouse, Denver, CO. 1988.

Snelling, Robert. *The Right Job.* Viking Penguin, Inc., New York, NY. 1987.

Stengel, Deborah. "Contract Physical Therapy Services: How to Provide Them," *Clinical Management.* American Physical Therapy Association, Alexandria, VA. 1987, No. 2:1-3.

Stengel, Deborah. "Contract Physical Therapy Services: The Wave of the Future?" *Clinical Management.* American Physical Therapy Association, Alexandria, VA. 1986, No. 6:4-6.

Stewart, Marjabelle; Faux, Marian, *Executive Etiquette.* St. Martin's Press, New York, NY. 1979.

Studner, Peter. *Super Job Search.* Jamenair LTD, Los Angeles, CA. 1987.

Tarrant, John. *Stalking the Headhunter: The Smart Job-Hunter's Guide to Executive Recruiters.* Bantam Books, Toronto, 1986.

Yoder, Dale; Staudohar, Paul. *Personnel Management and Industrial Relations.* Prentice-Hall, Englewood Cliffs, NJ. 1982.

INDEX

A

Advertisements: answering   45-47
    general tips of   109-110
    organizing campaign of   109
    types of   45-46
Advertising Agency   109
Answering Machine   92
Assistants: in organizational layout   102
    occupational therapy   117-118
    physical therapy   117-118
American Hospital Association Guide to Health
    Care Field   79, 167
American Journal of Occupational Therapy   44, 168
American Occupational Therapy Association   42, 117, 118
American Physical Therapy Association   42, 44, 117, 118
Application Form: filling out   84, 87
    sample of   85
Aptitude: general intelligence   126
Attitude: general   44, 145, 148
    while interviewing   126
    with recruiters   49

B

Benefits: fringe   115
    offering competitive   89, 110
Bonuses: sign-on   112, 115

C

Career Fairs   113
Career Quiz   34
Checklist: employee concerns   114-115
    job search   157-158
Clinical Management   44, 104, 111, 115, 150, 168
College Placement Services   40
Communications: with the interview   86
    in strategies of staffing   100, 104
Contracting Companies   115-116

Conventions   42
Cover Letters: pointers for   38, 47, 53-54
    sample   55-63

D

Directories   167
Discrimination: dealing with, in hiring   131
    in advertisements   109
Dressing: for the interview   81, 87
Drinking: at meals   88

E

Education: clinical education programs   111
    continuing   90, 138
    interview discussion of   126
    programs   110, 115
    scholarships and stipends   111
    teaching   111
    work study   111-112
Employment Agencies   47-49, 113
Employment History   125
Etiquette: post-interview   94
    with termination   140-141
Examination: national   117
    self   147
    state   117
Expenses: with interviewing and relocation   89-114

F

Financing: methods of   79
Food: eating difficult   88
Forcasting: future staffing needs   104
Friends   42, 148

G

Geographical Considerations   28-30, 38
Goals: developing   22, 157

H

Healthcare Delivery: components of   79
Hiring Decision   121, 128

Hospitals   39, 168
Housing: provided for   112

I

Immigration and Naturalization Service   113
Institute of Medicine   13
International Recruitment   113
Interviews: definition   77
    detailed topics of   125-126
    etiquette after   94, 158
    factors of employee concern at   114
    letters sent after   94-96
    positives and negatives of job   87
    questions at   88-92
    steps in   78-88
    telephone manners with   92-93
    tricky questions at   90-92

J

Job Change Reasons   30-32
Job Description: functions of   106, 149, 151
    in interview questions   89
    sample   107-108
    with contract negotiations   116
Job Offer: Letter of confirmation   131
    sample letter declining   96
    sample letter of   130
Job Sharing   105
Journal of American Physical Therapy
    Association   *139, 44, 169*

L

Language: addressing interviewer   84
    misused words   86
    with interview   84, 86
    with telephone   92-93
Law: legal requirements   109, 131-132
    pre-employment inquiry guide   132, 134-137
    with termination   141
Leters: cover   38, 47, 53-63

sample offer   130
    thank-you   94-96, 158
Libraries: researching job search   39, 41, 78-79
License: application form   85
    in confirming employment   126
Listening   86-87
Logs: personal   161
    phone   162
    mail   163
    interview   164
    follow-up   165
    responses-offers/acceptances/rejections   166

M

Mail: use of in advertising campaign   109
Management: contract   115-117
    practices   91, 100-104
Meals: during interviews   86, 88

N

Names: use of first   84
National Center for Health Statistics   13
National Easter Seal Society   30, 168
Networking: during the search   41, 43
    post-search   146-147
Newspapers: advertising   45-47, 109-110
    resources as   167
    spotting news in   147

O

Occupational Outlook Handbook   14, 80
Occupational Therapy Assistants   102, 117-118
Occupational Therapy Forum   39, 147, 159, 169
Occupational Therapy Week   39, 169
Older American Act   13
Open House   113
Organizations   167-168
Organizational Layout Charts   102-103
Orientation: employee   132-133

P

Patients: types   14, 28, 80, 89, 91, 114
    with family centered model   103
Performance Review: purpose of   100, 138, 151
    sample of   139
Periodicals   39, 168-169
Personality   87, 126
Personnel or Human Resources Department   78, 101
Physical Therapy Assistants   102, 117-118
Physical Therapy Bulletin   39, 112, 169
Physical Therapy Forum   39, 160, 169
Physical Therapy/Occupational Therapy
    Job News   139, 169
Planning: steps in job search   37-39
Pre-Employment Inquiry Guide: lawful   134-137
    unlawful   134-137
Professional Contacts   41-43
Promotion or Transfer   24, 105
Publications   39, 43-44, 167-169

Q

Questions: lawful   134-137
    to answer during interview   90-92
    to ask during interview   88-90
    unlawful   134-137
Quiz: therapists' career   34

R

Radio-TV
    advertising campaign   109
    with networking   147
Recordkeeping Requirements   132
Reference: checking   38, 127-128
    form   129
Rehabilitation Department: modern department of   103
    traditional organization layout of   102
Relocation: in employee concerns   114
    in interview questions   89
    in strategies of staffing   112

179

with employment agencies   48
with geographical consideration   29-32
Replacement Planning   104
Resources: for job openings advertising   39, 167-169
    directories as   167
    newspapers as   39,167
    organizations as   167-168
    periodicals as   168-169
Resumes: critique of   65
    sample   66-73
    writing   64-65
Risks and Gains   28

S

Salary: obtaining   149-151
    offering competitive   110, 128
    surveys   159-160
Secretary: relationship with   83
Selection Process: checking references in   127-129
    final decision in   128
    interviewing in   123-126
    job offer in   128, 130-131
    ranking in   122-123
    screening in   122
Self Evaluation: quiz of   33-34, 147
    strenghts and weaknesses of   24-27, 38, 91
Shaking Hands   84, 87
Smoking   83, 87-88
Staffing Strategies: retention and recruitment in   99-118
Success: general tips of   147-149

T

Table Manners   88
Telephone: manners   92-93
    tips with advertisements   109-110
Termination: giving warning in   140
    legal issues of   141
    rules of etiquette with   140-141
Thank-You Letters: after interview   94-95, 158
    declining offer   96

Time: at interview arrival   82
      length of interview   123
Timetable: of job change   153-154
Today's Student Physical Therapist   39, 169
Travel: for interview   81-82, 87, 92
Treatment Procedures   89

U

Unpublished Market   40-41

W

Work Schedules   104-105, 115

ORDER BY MAIL

To order, complete the information below, enclose it in your envelope with a check or money order. Mail to:

THERAPY CAREERS PRESS
29451 Greenfield #112
Southfield, MI 48076

Name_____Title_____

Organization _____Telephone ( )_____

Street Address _____

City _____State_____Zip_____

1-4 books	$25.00 ea.	25-49 books	$20.00 ea.
5-14 books	$22.50 ea.	50-99 books	$18.75 ea.
15-24 books	$21.25 ea.	over 100 books	$17.50 ea.

Enclose check or money order for payment in full

_____ copies of *Physical & Occupational Therapists'*
Job Search Handbook

at $_____ each $ _____

Michigan residents add 4% sales tax $ _____

Shipping and Handling add $3.50
(plus $.75 per book for orders of
  2 or more) $ _____

                        TOTAL $ _____

182